Safe Filler Injection Techniques

Won Lee

Safe Filler Injection Techniques

An Illustrated Guide

Funder not in Funder Registry

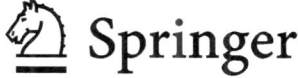 Springer

Won Lee
Yonsei E1 Plastic Surgery Clinic
Anyang, Kyonggi-do, Korea (Republic of)

1ˢᵗ edition: © MDWORLD Medical Publishing Co. 2021
ISBN 978-981-16-6854-8   ISBN 978-981-16-6855-5   (eBook)
https://doi.org/10.1007/978-981-16-6855-5

This Springer imprint is published by the registered company Springer Nature Singapore Pte Ltd. The registered company address is: 152 Beach Road, #21-01/04 Gateway East, Singapore 189721, Singapore

Minimal invasive techniques are based on clinical anatomy. Previously, anatomy was one of the essential medical subjects, but nowadays anatomy has evolved to be the basis of clinical procedures. A successful clinical result comes from understanding complex anatomical knowledge and its relationship with complications.

This book is based on recent science-based articles and clinical experiences. For beginners, it describes each procedure by photo illustration. It provides clinical indications from clinical anatomical illustrations and profound anatomical knowledge. There is no doubt, safe filler injections can be performed with the help of this book.

—Hee-Jin Kim, *Professor Yonsei University, Republic of Korea*

Aesthetic surgery is the combination of art and science, and while you cannot gauge the "ART" part, you definitely can measure the "SCIENCE" part by the number of medical articles.

Of all the plastic surgeons I know, Dr. Lee is one of the best. His dedication to detail and knowledge about filler is unparalleled.

—Jin Liang Lee, MD, *Justmake Plastic Surgery, Taipei, Taiwan*

Congratulations on another big success and thanks for your efforts. This book will be the bible of filler injectors because it includes an organization of Dr. Lee's scientific research. Many doctors will be helped by this filler injector knowledge. Thanks again for providing abundant scientific-based true knowledge.

—Hyoung-Jin Moon, MD, IMCAS, *Scientific Faculty, Republic of Korea*

Congratulations to Dr. Won Lee on the publication of this new Guidebook of Filler Injection. The Guidebook will be a valuable resource for all who wish to achieve the safest and best outcomes from fillers.

—Hema Sundaram, MD, FAAD, *Board Certified Dermatologist, USA*

"Won Lee." He is not a good speaker. He does not have a sense of humor nor does he give a long-winded explanation. He never minces his words. He always talks specifics and expresses himself truly.

He wrote about his clinical experience and research in this book using clean words and honesty. His passion is shown in each sentence of the book. It is of great fortune that he is with us.

—Wook Oh, MD, *President ICLAS, Republic of Korea*

Soft tissue augmentation has been in existence for nearly 20 years and has become a popular procedure in many dermatologic and plastic surgery practices. When used properly, fillers injection can be used to treat a wide range of different conditions—from filling lines and grooves on the face to facial contouring. It is imperative that practitioners understand the science of fillers and injection techniques in order to deliver safe and effective treatment.

In his book, *Safe filler injection; An illustrated Guide,* Dr. Won Lee provides insight into different injection techniques for each individual patient and treated area. The illustrative tables and "before and after" treatment photos enable readers to not only appreciate the changes that can result from these different techniques, but also provides them with important information for the formulation of treatment plans specific to their own patients.

—Rungsima Wanitphakdeedecha, M.D., M.A., M.Sc., *Faculty of Medicine Siriraj Hospital, Mahidol University, Bangkok, Thailand*

Dr. Won Lee is one of the leading scholars and world-class plastic surgeons on injectables in the world. He devotes himself not only to clinical practices and research, but also medical education and publications. His publications focusing on clinical anatomy and injection techniques are of high contribution to the enhanced standards of clinical practices and injectables safety. We are both partners in delivering lectures to educating practitioners around the world. His articles and talks are always very informative and inspiring. I appreciate very much his strong support for medical education.

I believe this new book will benefit all practitioners in aesthetic medicine and soon, people all around the world. I look forward to his next new publications. Best wishes in his work to improve injectables practices and education.

—Patrick Huang, MD, FAADV, *Expert in Dermatology and Skin Surgery, Taiwan*

I have known Dr. Won Lee from several international conferences and he has been an avid speaker with frequent academic publications. When I heard about his new book on how to inject Hyaluronic Acid Fillers, I was thrilled to be writing a recommendation for him. With his knowledge and experience in the artistry of injectology, I am sure this book will be a great reference and learning tool for our industry and also doctors keen on learning how to do fillers in a much safer and effective way. This is a book that every injector should not miss!

—Tingsong Lim, MD, *Clique Clinic, Kuala Lumpur, Malaysia*

As an educator, I endeavor to stay at the forefront of fast evolving and evidence-based practices in aesthetic medicine. There are so many books in the field of facial injectables, yet it can be quite challenging for the beginner or advanced aesthetic physician, to up-skill, stay current and improve patient outcomes, safely.

I found this book to provide simple yet comprehensive scientific insights into safe injection techniques, product choice, and anatomy for the whole face.

It is my pleasure to highly recommend this excellent, practical, and clinically relevant book.

—Sabrina Shah-Desai, MD, MS, FRCS, *Director Perfect Eyes Ltd & Oculo-Facial Aesthetic Academy (OFAA), London, UK*

Preface

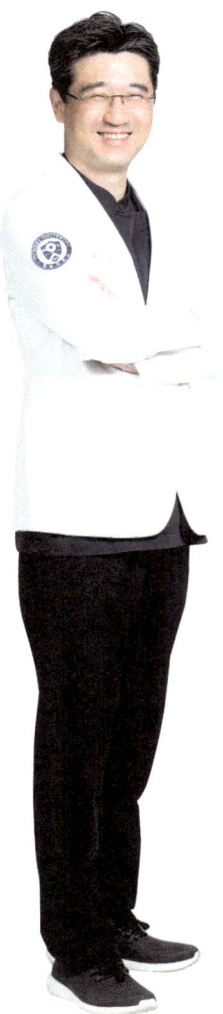

A filler injection is called a blind procedure because you cannot see everything under the surface. So there is no right answer for the injection technique. But definitely there are some injection techniques that should not be performed because of their direct relation to complications. There seem to be a few articles that suggest injection techniques that I believe should not be performed. And so, through this guide, I want to organize recommended techniques supported by scientific evidences. I especially wish to guide beginners using illustrated photographs with the hopes of wrong techniques not being performed.

I have written 40 SCI articles thus far and each one offers precious insight into safe injection practice. While I have written many articles about filler injection techniques, I have yet to find the right answer. But imagine if the patient in front of you is your daughter, you should perform the safest scientific procedure possible.

As I described, I want to show safe techniques step by step. I also want to show each technique supported by scientific evidences. It is my wish that all injectors in the world will be reminded of the safe injection techniques and that no complications develop.

To publish this book, I would like to offer special thanks to Yeo Myeung Yoon for your great support.

And as always, I give thanks to Seung Hyun, Hyun Ji, and Jung Youn with love.

Anyang Kyonggi-do, South Korea   Won Lee

Contents

Won Lee is a plastic surgeon. He received his MD from Yonsei University Medical College and PhD from College of Medicine, Dongguk University, Seoul, South Korea. Currently, he is the Director of Yonsei E1 Plastic Surgery Clinic, Anyang.

Dr. Lee is a member of the Korean Society of Plastic and Reconstructive Surgeons and a member of the Minimal Invasive Plastic Surgery, South Korea. He wrote "Filler Complications" from Spring 2019. He wrote various articles about filler injection and those are as follows:

1. Novel technique of filler injection in the temple area using the vein detection device JPRAS 2018

2. Practical Guidelines for Hyaluronic Acid Soft-Tissue Filler Use in Facial Rejuvenation. Dermatol Surg 2019

3. Effectiveness of retrobulbar hyaluronidase injection in an iatrogenic blindness rabbit model using hyaluronic acid filler injection. PRS 2019

4. Nasal dorsum augmentation using soft tissue filler injection. JCD 2019

5. Soft tissue properties can be altered by a small diameter Dermatol Surg 2019

6. Ocular complications of soft tissue filler injections: A review of literature JCD 2019

7. Comments on "Update on Avoiding and Treating Blindness From Fillers: A Recent Review of the World Literature" ASJ 2020

8. Comparative Effectiveness of Different Interventions of Perivascular Hyaluronidase PRS 2020

9. Safe Doppler ultrasound-guided method for nasolabial fold correction with hyaluronic acid filler ASJ 2020

10. Prevention of hyaluronic acid filler-induced blindness IMCAS letter, Dermatologic therapy 2020

11. Comments on "Filler rhinoplasty based on anatomy: The dual plane technique" JPRAS 2020

12. Safe Glabellar Wrinkle Correction With Soft Tissue Filler Using Doppler Ultrasound ASJ 2020

13. Development and Usability of a Virtual Reality-Based Filler Injection Training System APS 2020

14. Doppler Ultrasonographic Anatomy of the Midline Nasal Dorsum APS 2020

15. Identification of a suitable layer for injecting calcium hydroxyapatite fillers in the hands JPRAS 2020

16. Comments on "Hyaluronidase: an overview of its properties, applications, and side effects" Archive PS 2020

17. Comparison of hyaluronic acid filler ejection pressure with injection force for safe filler injection JCD 2021

18. Aspiration revisited: Prospective evaluation of a physiologically pressurized model with animal correlation and broader applicability to filler complications ASJ 2021

19. Unexpected Bone Resorption in Mentum Induced by the Soft-Tissue Filler Hyaluronic Acid: A Preliminary Retrospective Cohort Study of Asian Patients PRS 2021

20. Aspiration Before Filler Injection: Rethinking the Paradigm? ASJ 2021

The most tragic filler complications are skin necrosis and ocular complications. Prevention is most important and is described in the article of *Dermatologic Therapy* (Fig. 1.1, Table 1.1).

1.1 (An) Anatomy (Doppler Ultrasound)

Anatomical knowledge is most important for prevention. In particular, injectors should be aware of the important vessels of the face (Fig. 1.2).

Internal carotid artery branches: Supratrochlear artery, supraorbital artery, and dorsal nasal artery.

External carotid artery branches: Superficial temporal artery, facial artery, and infraorbital artery.

Knowing anatomy is the most important element in prevention but injectors are incapable of knowing all the variations of the vessels. So recently, using a Doppler ultrasound for detecting arteries before filler injection, has been proposed (Fig. 1.3).

1.2 Doppler Ultrasound Detection of Important Arteries of the Face

(1) Supratrochlear artery.

This chapter describes the relationship between glabellar wrinkles and the supratrochlear artery. To correct the glabellar wrinkle line, it is common to inject hyaluronic acid filler (Fig. 1.4). But one of the most common sites of ocular complication is correcting the glabellar wrinkle line [3]. This is because it is common that the supratrochlear artery tends to be located just beneath the glabellar wrinkle line and it is possible to inject into the ophthalmic artery.

It is safe to inject at the glabellar wrinkle lines if the supratrochlear artery is located in another site (Fig. 1.5) but it is impossible to inject filler to the glabellar wrinkle line if the supratrochlear artery is located at the glabellar wrinkle lines (Fig. 1.6).

(2) Dorsal nasal artery.

When we perform injection rhinoplasty, it is essential to know the dorsal nasal artery location. But the dorsal nasal artery has many variations and in many cases the artery crosses the midline (Fig. 1.7). In such cases, when performing an injection at the midline, a vascular complication might occur.

This chapter describes dividing the nose by radix, rhinion, supratip, and tip. In many cases, the intercanthal veins are located at the radix and the dorsal nasal arteries are located at the rhinion (Fig. 1.8).

It is relatively safe to use a cannula but it is not 100% safe. The dorsal nasal artery has variations and in some rare cases, the artery is detected at the supraperiosteal layer (Fig. 1.9). The most

Received: 26 March 2020 | Revised: 2 May 2020 | Accepted: 17 May 2020

DOI: 10.1111/dth.13657

IMCAS: LETTER

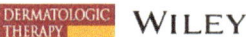

Prevention of hyaluronic acid filler-induced blindness

Fig. 1.1 Prevention of HA filler—Dermatologic Therapy 2020 [1]

Table 1.1 ABCs in the prevention of filler-induced ocular complications

(An) Anatomy (Doppler ultrasound)
(As) Aspiration with proper technique
(B) Big cannulas
(C) Compression
(D) Direction of injection
(E) Emergency kit
(F) Filler technique for augmentation or wrinkle correction
(G) Gentle injection of a small amount
(H) History of prior operations or injections

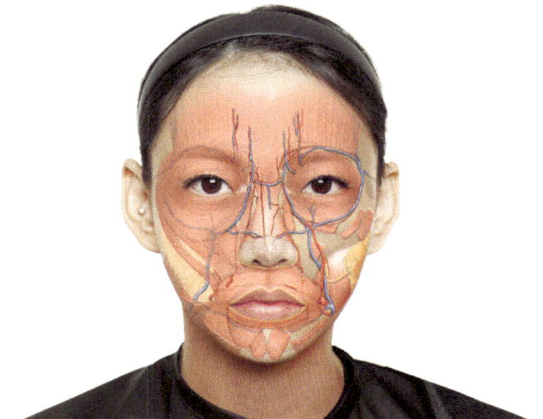

Fig. 1.2 Important vessels of the face

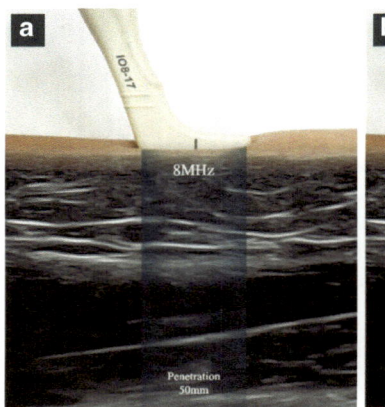
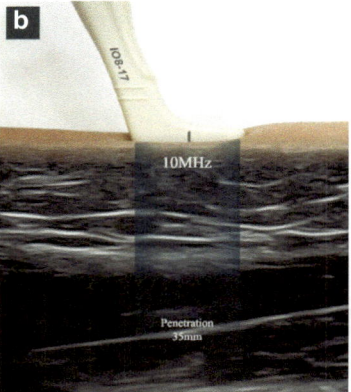
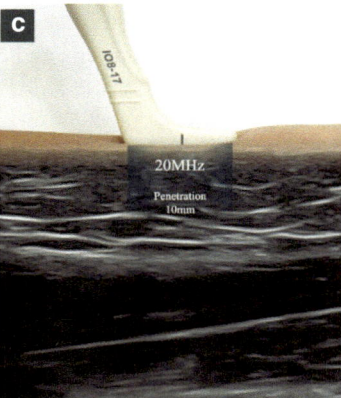

Fig. 1.3 The depth relationship within ultrasound frequency. Between 8 and 10 MHz frequency is mostly used in plastic surgery fields. (**a**) Within 8MHz frequency, 50mm depth can be detected. Most of the facial layer can be detected. (**b**) Within 10MHz frequency, 35mm depth can be detected. (**c**) Within 20MHz frequency, 10mm depth can be detected. Dermal layer can be seen precisely

common location of ocular complication was found to be injections at the nose [6]. Injection rhinoplasty is the easiest and most efficient way of nonsurgical rhinoplasty but should be performed very carefully.

(3) Facial artery.

The nasolabial fold correction is one of the most performed filler injections. The facial artery runs under the mimetic muscle or over the mus-

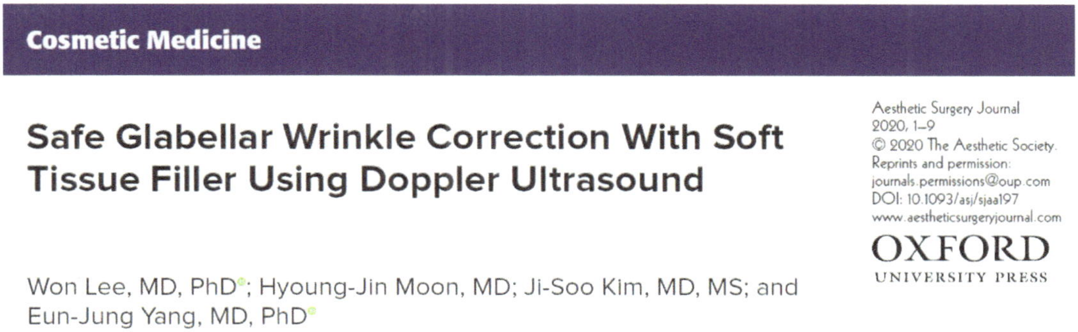

Cosmetic Medicine

Safe Glabellar Wrinkle Correction With Soft Tissue Filler Using Doppler Ultrasound

Aesthetic Surgery Journal
2020, 1–9
© 2020 The Aesthetic Society.
Reprints and permission:
journals.permissions@oup.com
DOI: 10.1093/asj/sjaa197
www.aestheticsurgeryjournal.com

OXFORD
UNIVERSITY PRESS

Won Lee, MD, PhD°; Hyoung-Jin Moon, MD; Ji-Soo Kim, MD, MS; and
Eun-Jung Yang, MD, PhD°

Fig. 1.4 Glabellar wrinkle correction by filler injection [2]

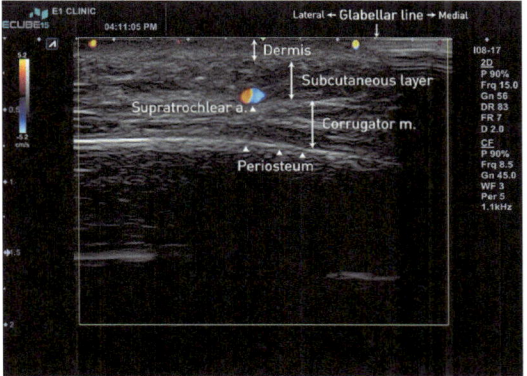
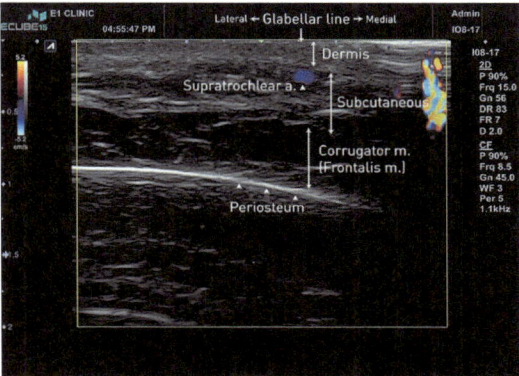

Fig. 1.5 Doppler ultrasound finding of glabellar wrinkle line. The supratrochlear artery's location is lateral from the glabellar wrinkle line

Fig. 1.6 Doppler ultrasound finding of glabellar wrinkle line. The supratrochlear artery is located at the subdermal layer just beneath the glabellar wrinkle lines

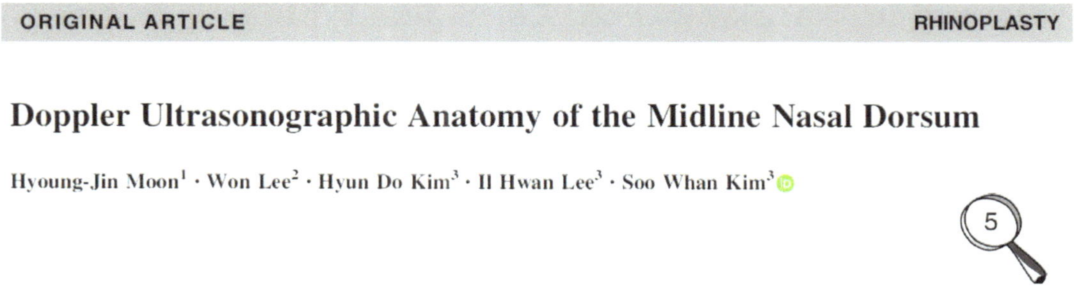

ORIGINAL ARTICLE   **RHINOPLASTY**

Doppler Ultrasonographic Anatomy of the Midline Nasal Dorsum

Hyoung-Jin Moon[1] · Won Lee[2] · Hyun Do Kim[3] · Il Hwan Lee[3] · Soo Whan Kim[3]

Fig. 1.7 Doppler ultrasound article at *Aesthetic Plastic Surgery* 2020 [4]

cle [7]. When a facial artery embolism occurs, the lateral nasal artery can be obstructed and skin necrosis may develop in the nose alar area. When an embolism occurs at the angular artery and ophthalmic artery, the most tragic complication, the ocular complication, could occur. When performing a Doppler ultrasound at the nasolabial fold area (Fig. 1.10), the facial artery could not be detected (detoured branch of facial artery), but usually the subcutaneous location is found

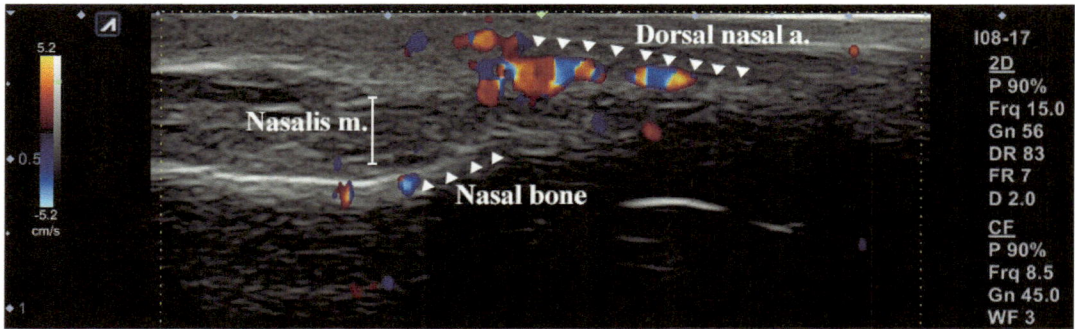

Fig. 1.8 Doppler ultrasound finding of the dorsal nasal artery at subcutaneous layer

ORIGINAL CONTRIBUTION

Nasal dorsum augmentation using soft tissue filler injection

Won Lee MD, PhD[1] | Ji-Soo Kim MD, MS[2] | Wook Oh MD[3] | Ik-Soo Koh MD, PhD[4] |
Eun-Jung Yang MD, PhD[5]

Fig. 1.9 Injection rhinoplasty by ultrasound in *Journal of Cosmetic Dermatology* (2019) [5]

Cosmetic Medicine

A Safe Doppler Ultrasound–Guided Method for Nasolabial Fold Correction With Hyaluronic Acid Filler

Aesthetic Surgery Journal
2020, 1–7
© 2020 The Aesthetic Society.
Reprints and permission:
journals.permissions@oup.com
DOI: 10.1093/asj/sjaa153
www.aestheticsurgeryjournal.com

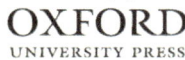

Won Lee, MD, PhD°; Ji-Soo Kim, MD, MS; Hyoung-Jin Moon, MD; and
Eun-Jung Yang, MD, PhD°

Fig. 1.10 Doppler ultrasound detection at nasolabial fold area. Published in *Aesthetic Surgery Journal* 2020 [8]

(Fig. 1.11). However, there are no safe places because there are some arteries in the deep medial cheek fat.

(4) Superficial temporal artery.

The frontal branch of the superficial temporal artery usually runs at the temple area along the hairline. So understanding the pathway is needed when performing a filler injection at the temple area or thread lifting. This artery is a relatively large diameter artery that can be detected easily by Doppler ultrasound (Fig. 1.12) [9].

There is a guideline of temple augmentation, which is injecting perpendicularly at 1 cm lateral and 1 cm above the lateral eyebrow [10]. But this technique might bring the risk of multiple vessels which are the superficial temporal artery, anterior

Fig. 1.11 Facial artery running at subcutaneous layer detected by Doppler ultrasound

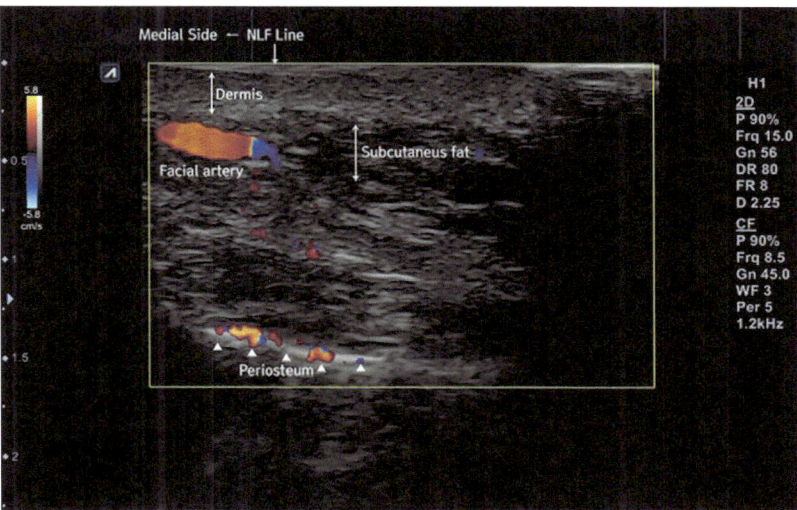

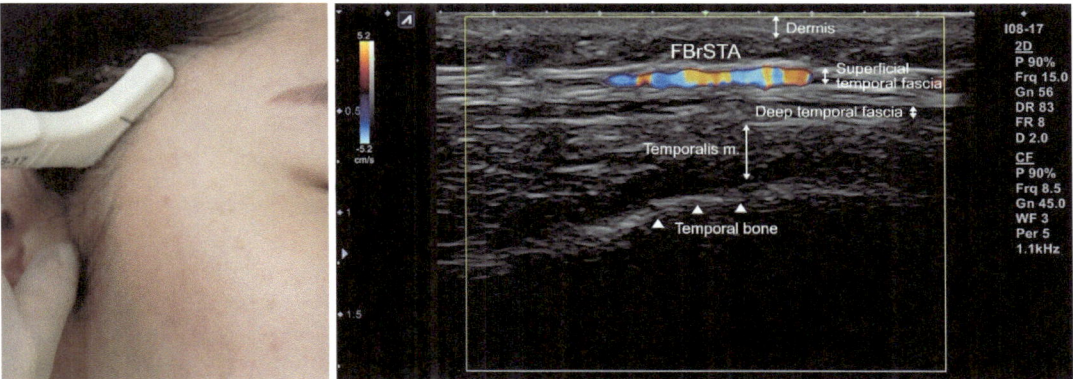

Fig. 1.12 Doppler ultrasound finding of frontal branch of superficial temporal artery

branch of deep temporal artery, zygomatico orbital artery, sentinel vein, and middle temporal vein (Fig. 1.13).

1.3 (As) Aspiration with Proper Technique

There are controversies about performing an aspiration test. Previous articles document false-negative findings by filler property, retraction, needle size, and so on. The author's finding was that a false negative is very much related to what substance is primed inside the needle (Fig. 1.14) [11].

The aspiration test is useless with the linear threading technique but is useful for the bolus injection technique. A false negative finding might occur by priming inside the needle, filler properties, the needle diameter, and so on.

1.4 (B) Big Cannula

All doctors agree that a cannula is safer than a needle. But we should be aware that a cannula is not 100% safe. A bigger diameter cannula is safer than a small diameter cannula. These are diagrams of comparison between common artery and cannula size (Fig. 1.15).

Fig. 1.13 Multiple arteries of temple area. A deep perpendicular needle injection brings risk to the superficial temporal artery or anterior branch of the deep temporal artery

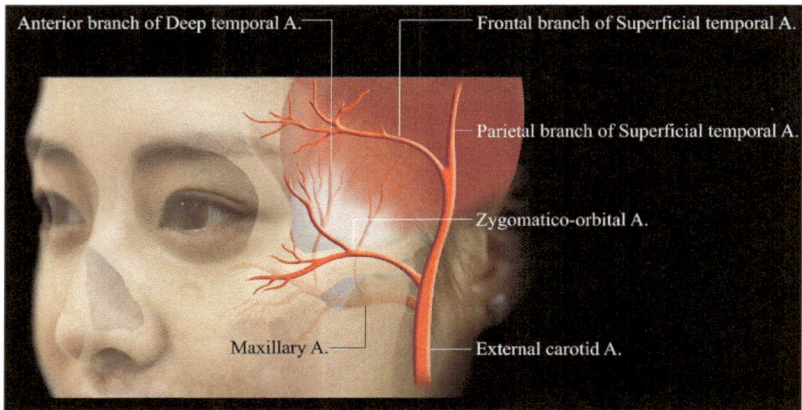

When performing compression and detection using the Doppler ultrasound, the artery is invisible (Fig. 1.17). Thus, compression could make filler penetrate into the artery.

So when performing a filler injection, it is recommended to use the opposite hand to compress the arterial pathway.

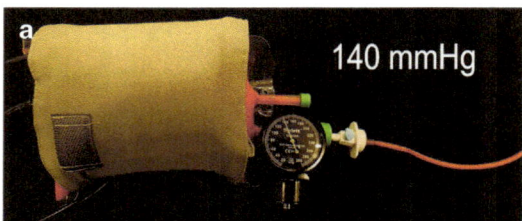

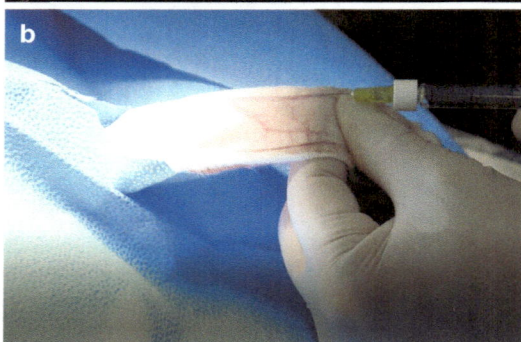

Fig. 1.14 Aspiration test. (**a**) In vitro (**b**) In vivo: an aspiration test performed on a rabbit femoral artery and central auricular vein

1.6   (D) Direction of Injection

The direction of the arterial pathway should be considered when undertaking a filler injection and it is relatively safe not to inject toward the eyes. For example, if a facial artery embolism occurs, it is better not to fill the embolism site toward the eye. This guideline is well explained by the ocular complication-induced nose filler injection. Many cases of ocular complication develop with the infralobular approach and embolism of the dorsal nasal artery. The infralobular approach is not a safe technique in the aspect of direction (Fig. 1.18).

1.5   (C) Compression

Compression during the injection and understanding the arterial pathway toward the ophthalmic artery is necessary. For example, compress the supratrochlear artery pathway when injecting at the glabellar area (Fig. 1.16).

1.7   (E) Emergency Kit

Filling is a relatively easy technique. But should a tragic complication such as skin necrosis or an ocular complication develop, both doctor and

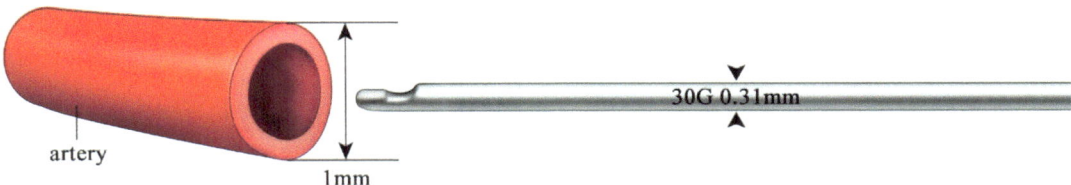

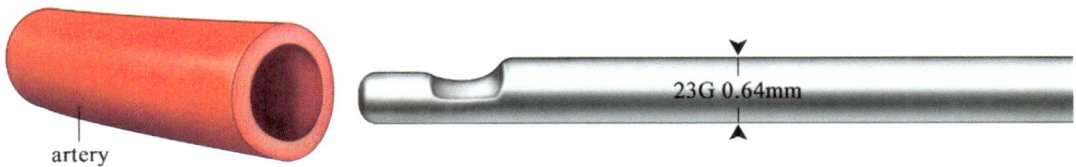

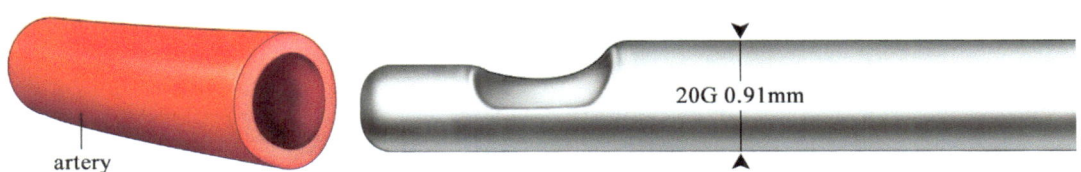

Fig. 1.15 The diameter of the important arteries (dorsal nasal artery, supratrochlear artery, and supraorbital artery) is approximately 1 mm diameter [12]. From the compara-tive diagram between arterial diameter and cannula, a relatively large diameter cannula cannot penetrate the artery

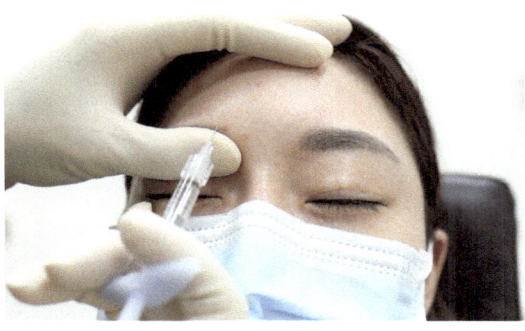

Fig. 1.16 Supratrochlear arterial pathway compression during glabellar wrinkle line correction

patient would panic. So, we should always pre-pare an emergency kit and mediate as soon as possible [13]. The author always prepares an emergency kit at the clinic (Fig. 1.19).

1.8   (F) Filler Techniques

The bolus technique is an effective technique for lifting tissue at a specific point. But we should inject a relatively large amount of volume. The aspiration test should be performed. In contrast, the linear threading technique moves the tip con-

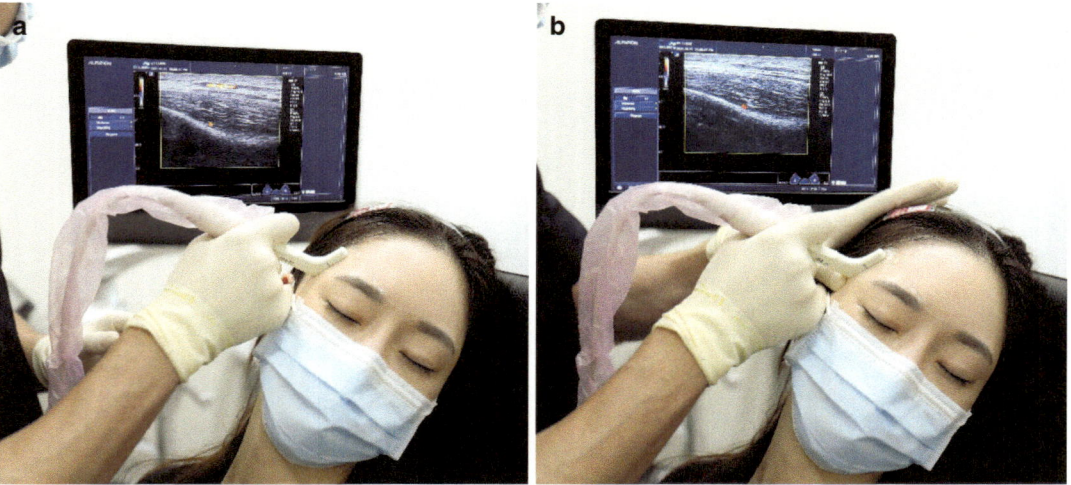

Fig. 1.17 (**a**) Superficial temporal artery detected by Doppler ultrasound. (**b**) Temple compression results in the artery disappearing

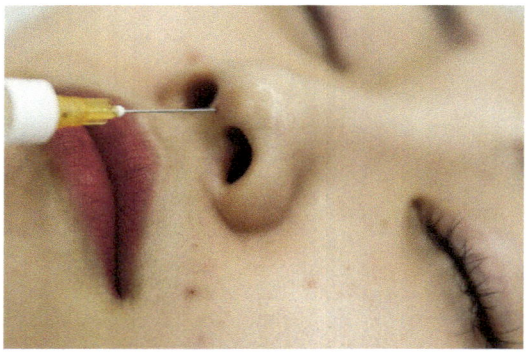

Fig. 1.18 Infralobular approach for nose filler injection. The cannula is heading toward the eye and this technique is not safe considering the direction of the injection. It is recommended to use a large diameter cannula and very gentle injection

tinuously and the aspiration test would seem useless. The injector should be aware of each injection technique for the prevention of complications.

1.9   (G) Gentle Injection of a Small Amount

The gentle injection is one of the most important factors of vascular complication. The chapter is about injection force and ejection pressure when performing hyaluronic acid filler injection (Fig. 1.20) [14].

Actual ejection pressure is much higher than normal blood pressure. This means the filler can reach the ophthalmic artery with a small injection force. A gentle injection with minimal force is needed (Fig. 1.21).

1.10   (H) History of Prior Operations or Injections

One preventive method is to ask about previous operation history or injection history. A previous operation would alter the vasculature. For example, the open rhinoplasty technique always interrupts the columellar artery and the nasal tip vasculature has to change. So extreme caution is needed for a previous operation site. The previous filler injection also might alter the vasculature. The vasculature might be compressed by previous filler injection and secondary injection space is decreased. Often we can find that the vascular complication occurs when performing a "retouching process."

Filler injection is a relatively simple technique. The patient needs a minimal invasive procedure for more aesthetic improvement and doctors also want to perform a minimal procedure. But there are some tragic complications and there are also no 100% safe techniques. But when performing a relatively safe procedure and per-

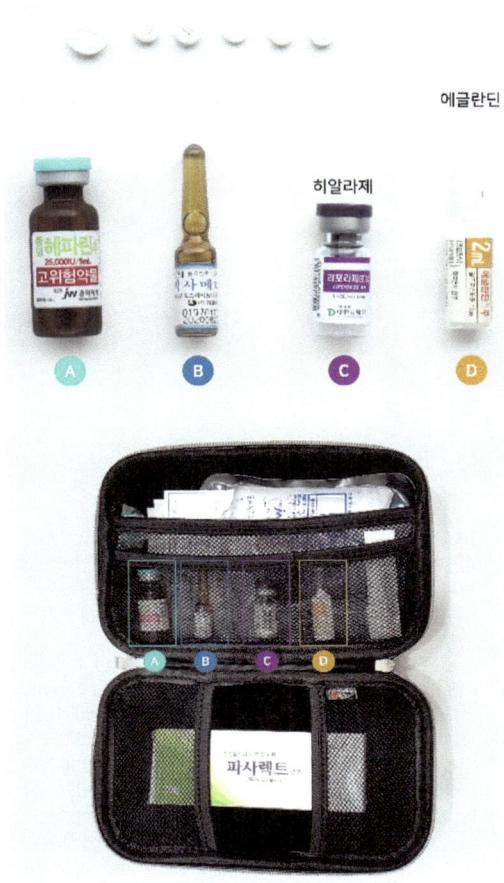

에글란딘

히알라제

Fig. 1.19   Emergency kit (A. Heparin, B. Dexamethasone, C. Hyaluronidase, D. E glandin)

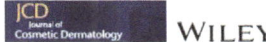 WILEY

ORIGINAL CONTRIBUTION

Comparison of hyaluronic acid filler ejection pressure with injection force for safe filler injection

Yongkoo Lee PhD[1] | Seung Min Oh MD, MMBA[2] | Won Lee MD, PhD[3] | Eun-Jung Yang MD, PhD[4]

Fig. 1.20   Pressure of hyaluronic acid filler injection

Fig. 1.21 The force of pushing filler out is called injection force and the actual pressure of the needle is called ejection pressure. Ejection pressure is calculated to be much higher than normal blood pressure

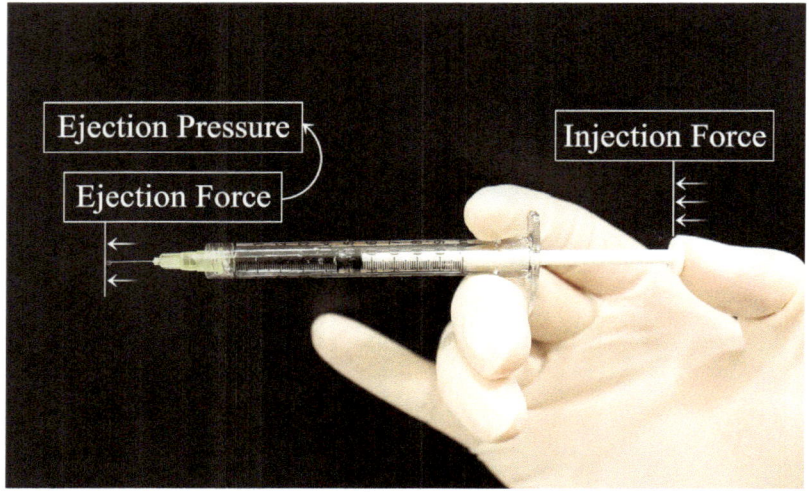

forming a repetitive safe procedure, a doctor would have a habit of injecting safely.

References

1. Lee W. Prevention of hyaluronic acid filler-induced blindness. Dermatol Ther. 2020 Jul;33(4):e13657. https://doi.org/10.1111/dth.13657. Epub 2020 Jun 23.
2. Lee W, Moon HJ, Kim JS, Yang EJ. Safe Glabellar Wrinkle correction with soft tissue filler using Doppler ultrasound. Aesthet Surg J. 2020;9:sjaa197. https://doi.org/10.1093/asj/sjaa197.
3. Beleznay K, Carruthers JD, Humphrey S, Jones D. Avoiding and treating blindness from fillers: a review of the world literature. Dermatol Surg. 2015 Oct;41(10):1097–117. https://doi.org/10.1097/DSS.0000000000000486.
4. Moon HJ, Lee W, Do Kim H, Lee IH, Kim SW. Doppler ultrasonographic anatomy of the midline nasal dorsum. Aesthet Plast Surg. 2021 Jun;45(3):1178–1183. https://doi.org/10.1007/s00266-020-02025-1. Epub 2020 Nov 2.
5. Lee W, Kim JS, Oh W, Koh IS, Yang EJ. Nasal dorsum augmentation using soft tissue filler injection. J Cosmet Dermatol. 2019 Jun 3; https://doi.org/10.1111/jocd.13018.
6. Beleznay K, Carruthers JDA, Humphrey S, Carruthers A, Jones D. Update on avoiding and treating blindness from fillers: a recent review of the world literature. Aesthet Surg J. 2019 May 16;39(6):662–74. https://doi.org/10.1093/asj/sjz053.
7. Lee JG, Yang HM, Choi YJ, Favero V, Kim YS, Hu KS, Kim HJ. Facial arterial depth and relationship with the facial musculature layer. Plast Reconstr Surg. 2015 Feb;135(2):437–44. https://doi.org/10.1097/PRS.0000000000000991.
8. Lee W, Kim JS, Moon HJ, Yang EJ. A safe Doppler ultrasound-guided method for nasolabial fold correction with hyaluronic acid filler. Aesthet Surg J. 2021 May 18;41(6):NP486–92. https://doi.org/10.1093/asj/sjaa153.
9. Lee W, Moon HJ, Kim JS, Chan BL, Yang EJ. Doppler ultrasound-guided thread lifting. J Cosmet Dermatol. 2020 Aug;19(8):1921–7. https://doi.org/10.1111/jocd.13240.
10. Swift A. One up, one over regional approach in "upper face: anatomy and regional approaches to injectables" found in the November 2015 supplement issue soft tissue fillers and neuromodulators: international and multidisciplinary perspectives. Plast Reconstr Surg. 2015;136:204S–18S.
11. Moon HJ, Lee W, Kim JS, Yang EJ, Sundaram H. Aspiration revisited: prospective evaluation of a physiologically pressurized model with animal correlation and broader applicability to filler complications. Aesthet Surg J. 2021 Apr 16:sjab194. https://doi.org/10.1093/asj/sjab194.
12. Choi DY, Bae JH, Youn KH, Kim W, Suwanchinda A, Tanvaa T, Kim HJ. Topography of the dorsal nasal artery and its clinical implications for augmentation of the dorsum of the nose. J Cosmet Dermatol. 2018 Aug;17(4):637–42. https://doi.org/10.1111/jocd.12720.
13. Prado G, Rodriguez-Feliz J. Ocular pain and impending blindness during facial cosmetic injections: is your office prepared? Aesthet Plast Surg. 2017;41(1):199–203.
14. Lee Y, Oh SM, Lee W, Yang EJ. Comparison of hyaluronic acid filler ejection pressure with injection force for safe filler injection. J Cosmet Dermatol. 2021 May;20(5):1551–6. https://doi.org/10.1111/jocd.14064.

Hyaluronic Acid Filler Property and Hyaluronidase

2

Hyaluronic acid is composed of disaccharides while hyaluronic acid filler is composed of a crosslinker and HA. This chapter will describe briefly the properties of hyaluronic acid filler and hyaluronidase.

2.1 Hyaluronic Acid Filler

Hyaluronic acid is a disaccharide structure (Fig. 2.1).

Hyaluronic acid filler is crosslinked between HA and HA by a crosslinker such as BDDE (1,4-butanediol diglycidyl ether, Fig. 2.2).

Depending on the manufacturing process, the amount of crosslinker is determined and is called the Modification of Degree (MOD). Usually, a biphasic filler's MOD is likely to be 1 ~ 3, compared to a monophasic filler at 5 ~ 10 and some filler's MOD is likely to be more than 10. But more important than the MOD is the actual crosslinked amount of BDDE, which is called the crosslinked MOD (cMOD) and pendant MOD (pMOD) (Fig. 2.3).

2.2 Rheology—First Parameter of Filler Property

Doctors should decide where and how to use new hyaluronic acid filler products (Fig. 2.4). Understanding is needed of such things as the

properties of the filler, how soft the injection will be, how hard the filler will be to lift the tissue and so on. These are some parameters to consider (Table 2.1).

It is determined to use a monophasic or biphasic filler at a specific area of the face. But doctors should determine their scientific knowledge and experience when choosing an appropriate HA filler. The author tested multiple HA filler products by his own rheometer to compare (Table 2.2).

Lorient 4 is similar to Restylane in terms of the rheometer results. When comparing these rheometer test results, doctors can estimate the filler product and determine the appropriate layer for injection. For example, with regard to the nasal and chin area, it is known that the supraperiosteal layer is a relatively safe layer for vascular complications but these two locations are compressed locations by muscle and a hard filler should be used to maintain the shape, such as Lorient No. 6.

2.3 Ideal Filler and Microscopic Finding

What is the ideal filler? According to previous literature, it is defined in Table 2.3.

Then what would be the HA filler (Fig. 2.5) for the ideal filler condition? It should be safe, biocompatible, and reversible. HA filler should be predictable and easy to use.

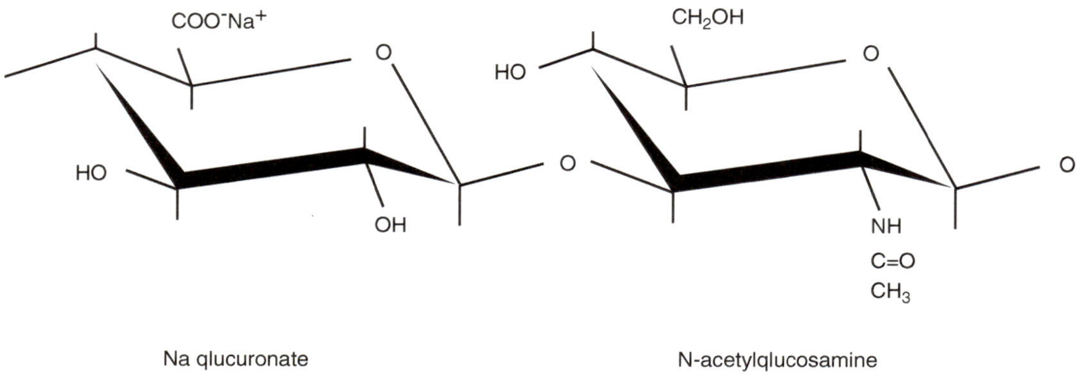

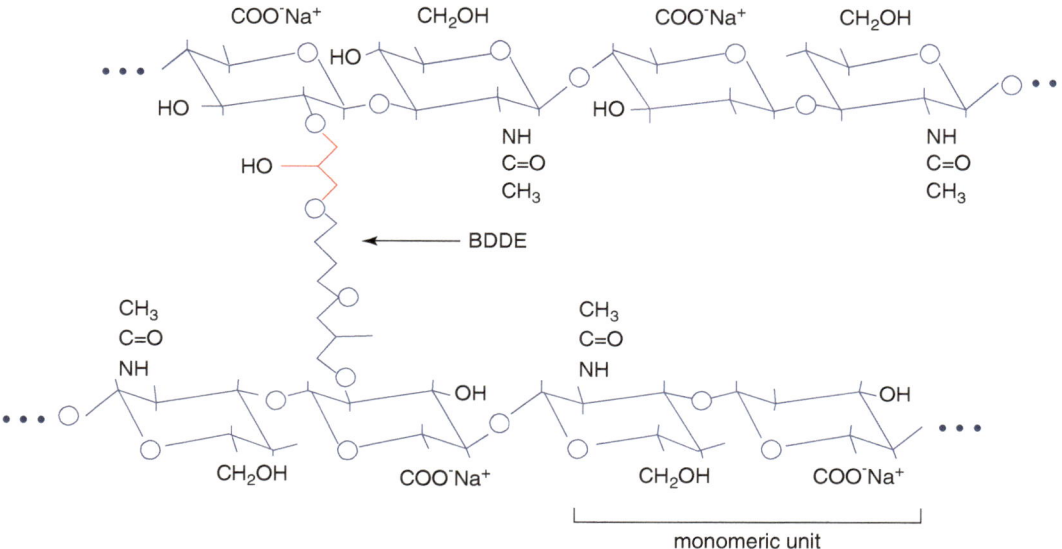

Fig. 2.1 Hyaluronic acid molecule

Fig. 2.2 Molecular structure of hyaluronic acid and crosslinker

Light microscopic findings and electron microscopic findings are as shown in Fig. 2.6.

Many preventive guidelines are suggested for vascular complications but changing the filler is not. But delayed hypersensitivity and formation of granuloma seem to be related to the filler product. Hyaluronic acid filler is a foreign body because there is a crosslinker inside the filler. But the immunologic reaction should be minimal. Although it is a foreign body, it should act as autologous tissue.

2.4   Hyaluronidase

The biggest advantage of using hyaluronic acid filler is that hyaluronidase can degrade the filler.

(1) Mechanism.

Generally, hyaluronidase dissolves hyaluronic acid, which exists in human tissue normally. It degrades β 1,4 chain of disaccharide (Fig. 2.7) (Leech hyaluronidase breaks β 1,3 chain).

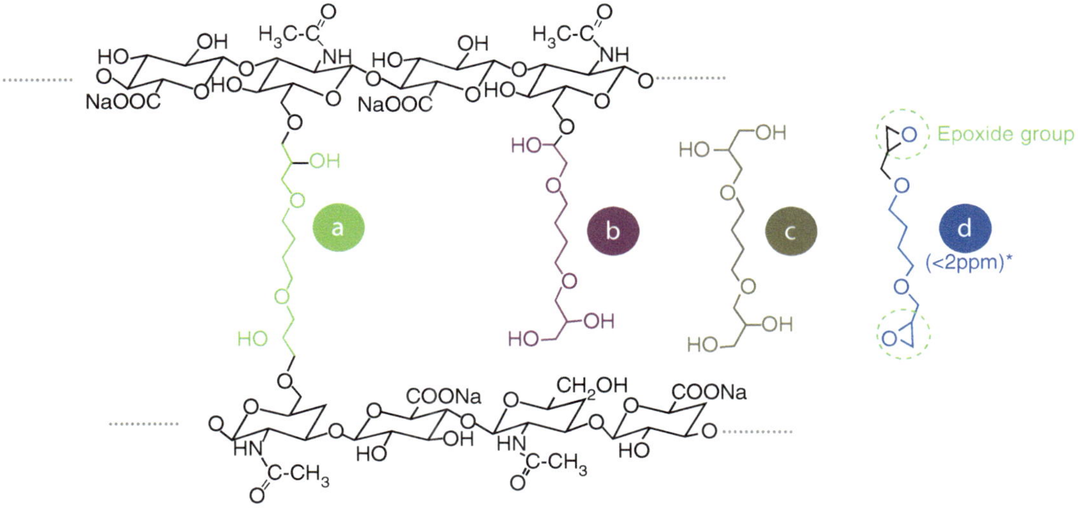

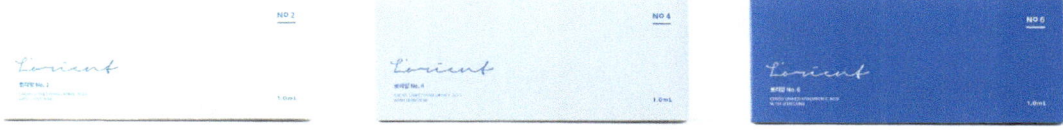

Fig. 2.3 Hyaluronic acid is crosslinked by BDDE. (**a**) Crosslinked, (**b**) Pendent, (**c**) Deactivated BDPE (1,4-butanediol di-(propan-2,3-diolyl) ether), and (**d**) Native

Fig. 2.4 Lorient HA filler (No. 2, No. 4, No. 6)

Table 2.1 Considerations when choosing HA filler

1. Manufacturing process—biphasic, monophasic.	Usually, biphasic filler has less cohesiveness and low MOD. BDDE and BDPE should be considered
2. Rheology results.	G', G'', G^*, cohesiveness [1]
3. Injection force.	When injection force is high, the risk is increased
4. Thixotrophy.	When injecting, filler should be soft After injection, filler is better to be hard enough to lift up the tissue
5. Crosslinked, pendent MOD.	Detectable by SEC/MS and complication is related to pendant type
6. Impurities.	Complication is directly related to impurities during manufacturing process (BDPE)
7. HA concentration.	Usually 20 mg/ml and is related to attaching adjacent water uptake

Table 2.2 Various HA fillers are tested by the author ((Frequency 0.02 Hz) MCR 301 rheometer (Anton Paar Co, Austria))

Product	G' (Pa)	G'' (Pa)	Complex viscosity (μ)	Tan delta	Cohesiveness (N)
Restylane	349	145	3,011,188	0.42	0.3509
Perlane	411	199	3,637,022	0.49	0.2869
Juvederm Voluma	284	58	2,309,805	0.21	0.4043
Lorient No 2	203	41	1,673,007	0.20	0.4401
Lorient No 4	338	95	2,795,776	0.28	0.4237
Lorient No 6	413	121	3,423,232	0.29	0.4454

At the dermal layer, there is abundant glycos-
aminoglycan including hyaluronic acid and hyaluronidase is used for hypodermoclysis. For
dissolving HA filler, hyaluronidase is usually off-
label use [3].

(2) Variety of hyaluronidase.

Hyaluronidase can be divided by manufacturing process, ovine testicular, bovine testicular, or

Table 2.3 Ideal filler [2]

- Non-toxic.
- Biocompatible.
- Long lasting (if not permanent).
- Reversible.
- Off the shelf.
- Autologous.
- Easy to use.
- Safe.
- Produces positive, natural, and discernible change.
- Minimal downtime.
- Level of placement (could be placed through
  dermis at subcutaneous, intramuscular, or
  periosteal level).
- Predictable.
- Performs well as a person ages.
- Not discernible by touch/appearance.

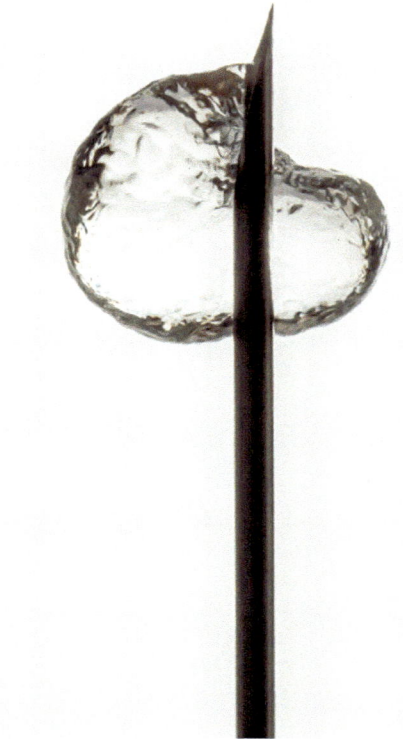

Fig. 2.5 Hyaluronic acid filler (Lorient)

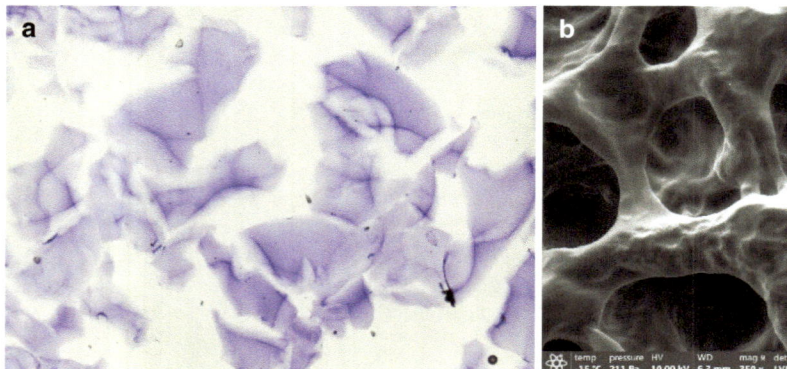
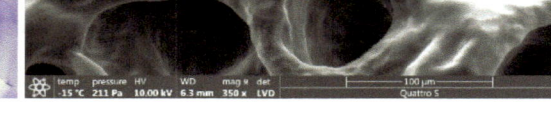

Fig. 2.6 Microscopic findings of hyaluronic acid filler. (**a**) Light microscopy and (**b**) Electron microscopy (Lorient)

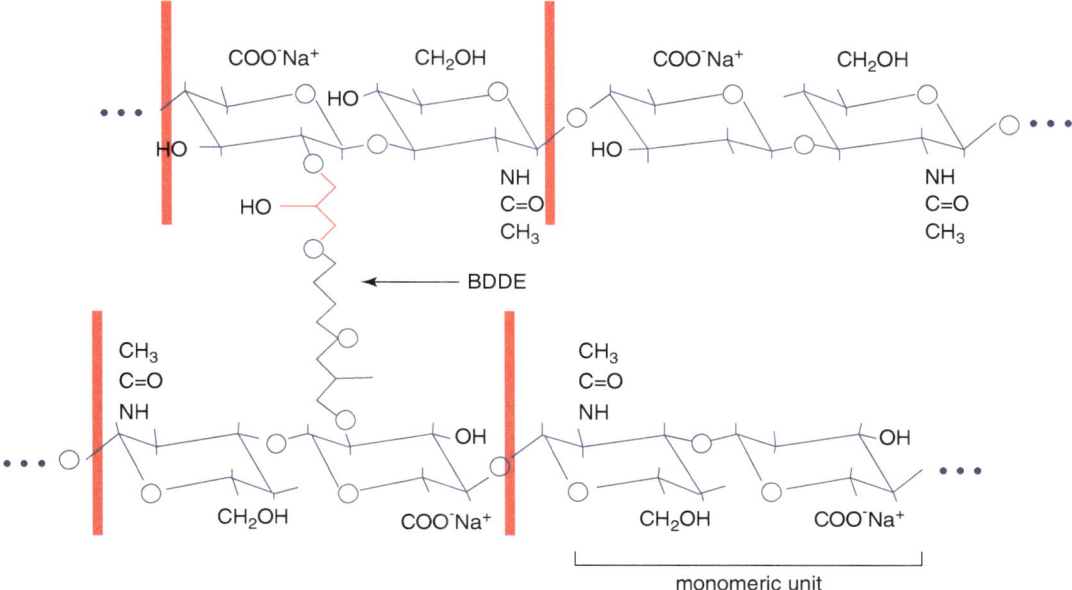

Fig. 2.7 Hyaluronidase breaks β 1,4 chain of disaccharides

human recombinant. Each product has different efficiency.

Also, there is a difference between countries. The United States usually uses Hylenex which is 150 USP and Vitrase which is 200 USP, while South Korea usually uses 1500 IU products (Fig. 2.8).

(3) Duration.

Hyaluronidase should be injected subcutaneously. The half-life of hyaluronidase is 30 mins in subcutaneous tissue and 2 ~ 3 mins in blood vessels. The theory of antibody formation in blood vessels is suggested.

(4) Nonvascular complication filler degradation.

A small amount of hyaluronidase can degrade nonvascular filler and result in complications such as nodules. The report shows

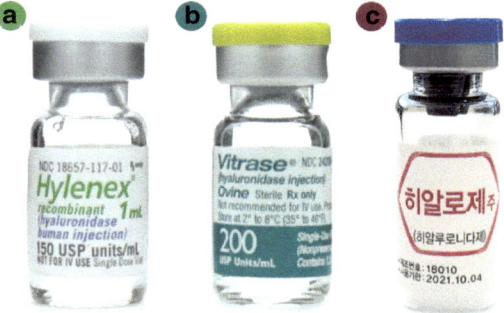

Fig. 2.8 Various types of hyaluronidase. (**a**) Hylenex 150 USP, (**b**) Vitrase 200 USP, and (**c**) Hyalose 1500 IU

30 ~ 60 IU to degrade in the animal model [4]. Also, there are reports that after 6 hours of hyaluronidase injection, the hyaluronic acid filler can be injected again [5]. So, a nodule can be degraded by a small amount. Granuloma already has a protective capsule so hyaluronidase might not degrade.

(5) Vascular complications.

The most tragic complication is a vascular complication. Doctors always prepare for vascular complications such as skin necrosis or ocular complications. Even though doctors are aware of vascular anatomy, there are always variations so it might occur with any patient.

What dose of Hyaluronidase should be injected?

Dr. Lorenzi proposed the dose of skin necrosis (Fig. 2.9) [6]. But multiple factors should be considered (Table 2.4).

Among these considerations, repetitive injections are very important. The author also conducted a rabbit experiment that found that an appropriate dose of hyaluronidase is needed and repetitive injections at 30 mins to 1 hour are needed [7].

Fig. 2.9 Dose for skin necrosis. The dose should be considered by various types of hyaluronidase product

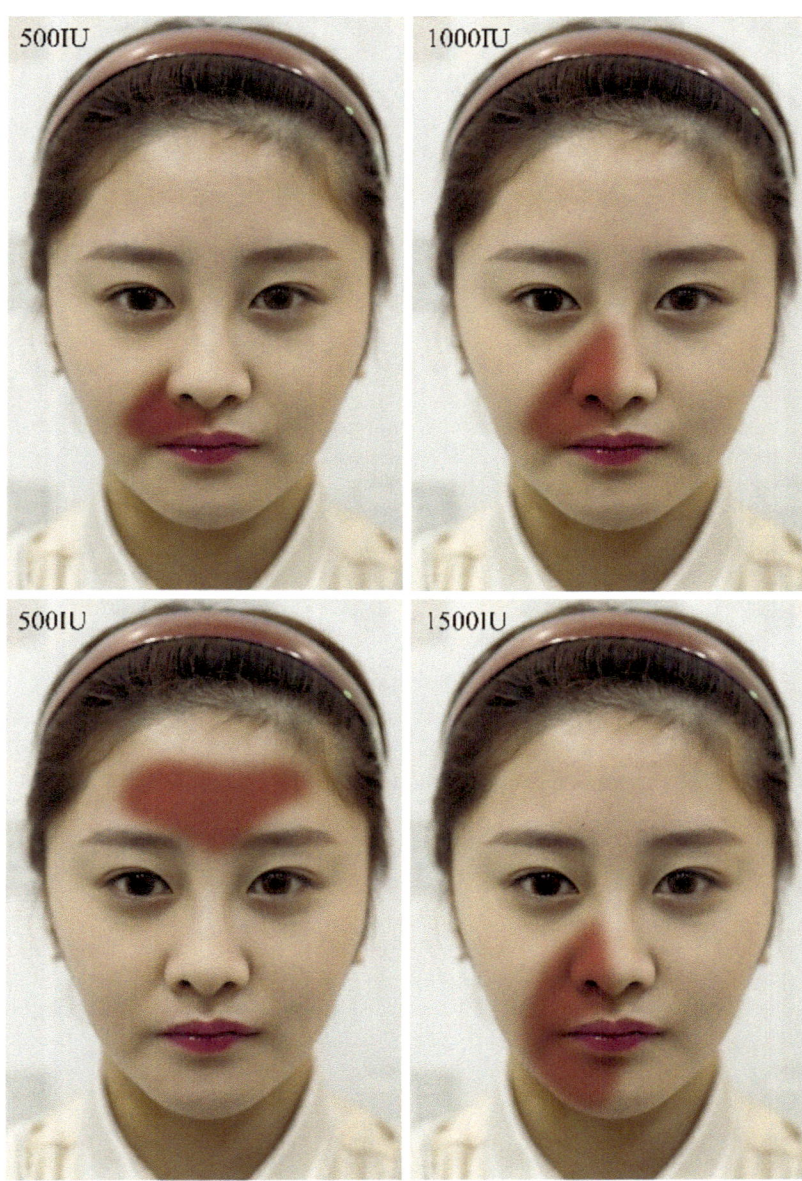

Table 2.4 Multiple considerations for hyaluronidase injection

1. Injected filler MoD.	HA fillers have a different degradation time because of a different MoD, BDDE, BDPE.
2. Efficiency of hyaluronidase.	Various types of hyaluronidase have different potencies.
3. Dose.	150, 200 USP are used in the United States, 1500 IU is often used in Korea.
4. Affected vessel.	Doctors should determine which vessels are involved and inject hyaluronidase as near as possible to the vessel but subcutaneously.
5. Degradation time.	Subcutaneously injected hyaluronidase cannot dissolve HA filler immediately.
6. Repetitive injection.	Subcutaneously injected hyaluronidase disappears when the half-life time passes. Repetitive injections are needed.

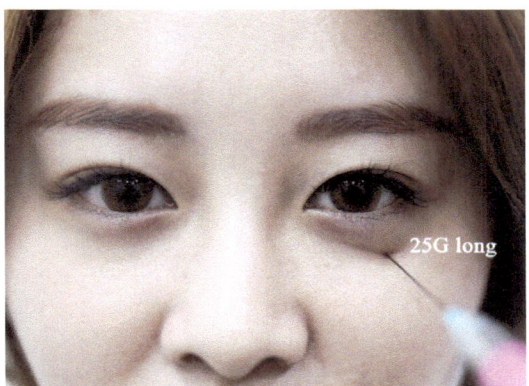

Fig. 2.10 Retrobulbar hyaluronidase injection [7]

(6) Ocular complication hyaluronidase.

Retrobulbar hyaluronidase injection has controversies (Fig. 2.10) [8] and other suggestive treatments are intraarterial injections [9], subtenon injections [10], and so on. This means the exact treatment is not revealed yet. Repetitive injections should also be considered and in the near future the treatment will be discovered.

References

1. Lee W, Hwang SG, Oh W, Kim CY, Lee JL, Yang EJ. Practical guidelines for hyaluronic acid soft-tissue filler use in facial rejuvenation. Dermatol Surg. 2020 Jan;46(1):41–9. https://doi.org/10.1097/DSS.0000000000001858.

2. Born TM, Airan LE, Suissa D. Injectables and resurfacing techniques: soft-tissue fillers. Rubin JP, Neligan PC, eds. Plastic surgery. Vol. 2 (2018): 39.

3. Lee W. Comments on "Hyaluronidase: an overview of its properties, applications, and side effects". Arch Plast Surg. 2020 Nov;47(6):626–7. https://doi.org/10.5999/aps.2020.01571.

4. Hwang E, Song YS. Quantitative correlation between hyaluronic acid filler and hyaluronidase. J Craniofac Surg. 2017 May;28(3):838–41. https://doi.org/10.1097/SCS.0000000000003411.

5. Kim HJ, Kwon SB, Whang KU, Lee JS, Park YL, Lee SY. The duration of hyaluronidase and optimal timing of hyaluronic acid (HA) filler reinjection after hyaluronidase injection. J Cosmet Laser Therapy. 2018;20(1):52–7.

6. DeLorenzi C. New high dose pulsed hyaluronidase protocol for hyaluronic acid filler vascular adverse events. Aesthet Surg J. 2017;37(7):814–25.

7. Lee W, Oh W, Oh SM, Yang EJ. Comparative effectiveness of different interventions of perivascular hyaluronidase. Plast Reconstr Surg. 2020 Apr;145(4):957–64. https://doi.org/10.1097/PRS.0000000000006639.

8. Lee W, Oh W, Ko HS, Lee SY, Kim KW, Yang EJ. Effectiveness of retrobulbar hyaluronidase injection in an iatrogenic blindness rabbit model using hyaluronic acid filler injection. Plast Reconstr Surg. 2019 Jul;144(1):137–43. https://doi.org/10.1097/PRS.0000000000005716.

9. Xu X, Zhou G, Fu Q, Zhang L, Yu Y, Dong Y, Liang L, Chen M. Efficacy of intra-arterial thrombolytic therapy for vision loss resulting from hyaluronic acid filler embolization. J Cosmet Dermatol. 2021 Apr 6; https://doi.org/10.1111/jocd.14111.

10. Choe HR, Woo SJ. Subtenon retrobulbar hyaluronidase injection for ophthalmic artery occlusion following facial filler injection. Int J Ophthalmol. 2020 Jul 18;13(7):1170–2. https://doi.org/10.18240/ijo.2020.07.25.

3.1 General Considerations

Oriental patients tend to have flat foreheads and prefer to have concave foreheads. The forehead is known to distinguish itself from the temple area by the superior temporal septum. But sometimes fillers tend to be injected across the superior temporal septum because of shape continuity. It is important to make a forehead shape by the doctor's aesthetic aspect and anatomical consideration.

In the anatomical aspect, the forehead has multiple layers such as skin, superficial fat, frontalis muscle, subgaleal space, and periosteum. The superficial fat layer is known to divide into the central forehead compartment and middle forehead compartment laterally. Clinically, a forehead depression is found at the central portion or lateral portion and this phenomenon is because of skull shape rather than volume of superficial fat. Usually, hyaluronic acid filler is injected at the subgaleal space known as the deep fat compartment [1].

It is important to consider the highest point because when a forehead is higher than the supraorbital ridge, the periocular region tends to appear sunken and the nasal area tends to appear relatively low (Fig. 3.1, Table 3.1). Also, when performing a nose augmentation, the doctor should consider the height of the forehead because the relationship between the forehead and nose is important.

Usually, a depressed area is shown between the frontal eminence and supraorbital ridge, so usually forehead augmentation by HA filler tends to be performed on this area. But this area is a dangerous location due to important vessel locations, so the filler injection should be performed very gently.

3.2 Anatomy

There are three main arteries in the forehead. These arteries are the supratrochlear artery, supraorbital artery, and frontal branch of the superficial temporal artery (Fig. 3.2).

The supratrochlear artery branches from the ophthalmic artery and runs from the medial part of orbit. It tends to run deeper than the layer of muscle and perforate the muscle to run superficially. The supraorbital artery runs with few variation patterns but usually runs in deeper portions and perforates muscle for superficial running. The supraorbital artery tends to make anastomosis with the frontal branch of the superficial temporal artery at the lateral sides of the forehead. Thus, it is very important for doctors to inject

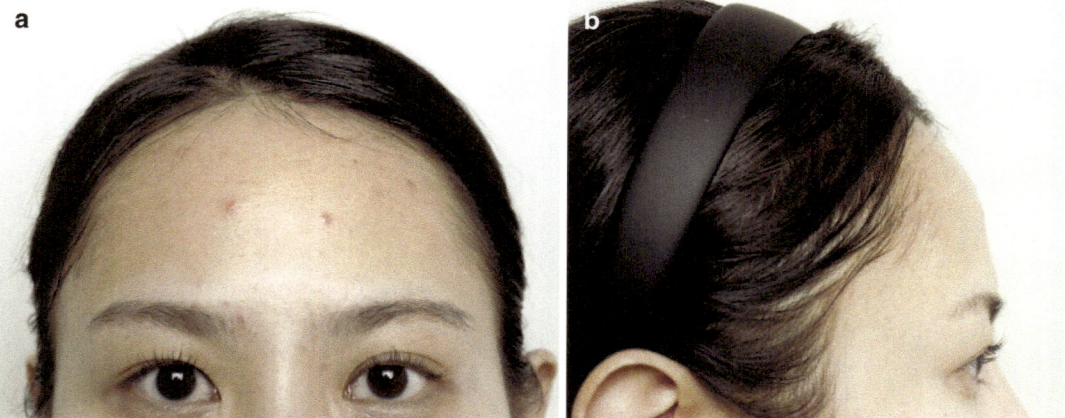

Fig. 3.1 Forehead considerations. (**a**) Front view and (**b**) Lateral view

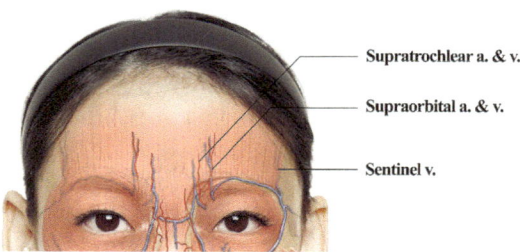

Supratrochlear a. & v.

Supraorbital a. & v.

Sentinel v.

Fig. 3.2 Forehead vessels

Table 3.1 Forehead considerations

Considerations of forehead augmentation by HA filler
1. The height of supraorbital ridge which is located near the eyebrow should be considered.
2. The highest desired location point of forehead should be considered.

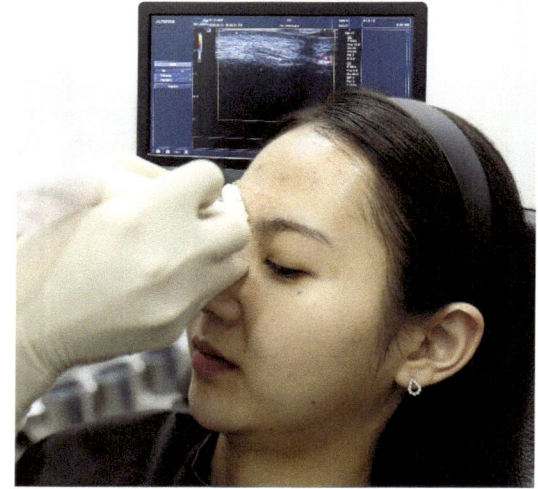

Fig. 3.3 Doppler ultrasound finding before forehead filler injection

gently and carefully when performing injections of HA filler deeply above the eyebrow, especially from eyebrow to 2 cm above.

3.3 Doppler Ultrasound

The superficial temporal artery is easily detected by the doppler ultrasound and the supratrochlear artery and the supraorbital artery can also be detected by ultrasound (Fig. 3.3). It is recommended to detect the supratrochlear artery and the supraorbital artery before any HA filler injection because these arteries are directly related to the ophthalmic artery [2].

3.4 Filler Choice

The forehead is a wide area so an even injection is quite important. Also, frontalis muscle action should be considered. Not only is the augmenta-

Table 3.2 The rheologic result of Lorient HA filler. The author prefers to use No. 4 for forehead augmentation

Product	G′ (Pa)	G″ (Pa)	Complex viscosity (μ)	Tan delta	Cohesiveness (N)
Lorient No. 2	203	41	1,673,007	0.20	0.4401
Lorient No. 4	338	95	2,795,776	0.28	0.4237
Lorient No. 6	413	121	3,423,232	0.29	0.4454

tion important but it should augment evenly and widely. Elasticity is important but cohesiveness is even more so when performing a forehead augmentation (Table 3.2).

3.5 Anesthesia

For a forehead augmentation, a topical anesthesia is not enough (Fig. 3.4), so a regional anesthesia is needed.

Regional anesthesia—The supratrochlear and supraorbital nerve anesthesia is performed (Fig. 3.5) but the lateral side of the forehead is innervated by the zygomaticotemporal nerve so doctors should also consider making a regional anesthesia at the zygomaticotemporal nerve.

3.6 Injection Layer

When we perform a forehead augmentation by implant, we should dissect under the periosteum and insert the implant. The dissection is not difficult but should be performed as bone scratching by a periosteal dissector. But when we perform a filler injection by cannula, it is almost impossible to dissect under the periosteum. Perpendicular injections by needle also cannot dissect under the periosteal layer. So most injected fillers tend to be located at the supraperiosteal layer [3]. A recent article also describes that it is impossible to inject filler at the subperiosteal layer, so the target layers for forehead injections should be the subgaleal layer or superficial fat layer [4].

When considering the arteries of the forehead, it is safer to inject at the subgaleal layer rather than the superficial fat layer. Usually, the supratrochlear artery and supraorbital artery tend to run superficially but just after a notch perforation

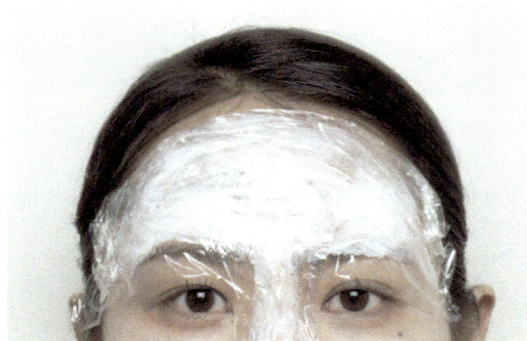

Fig. 3.4 Topical anesthesia is applied

they run at the subgaleal plane so extreme caution is needed near the eyebrow.

There is a central forehead compartment and middle forehead compartment at the forehead superficial fat layer and the superior temporal septum is located between the middle forehead compartment and lateral temporal cheek fat compartment [5]. Another reason for not injecting filler into the superficial fat layer is that septum can interrupt the injected filler spreading and irregularity can occur, so it is better to inject at the subgaleal plane.

3.7 Needle vs Cannula

A needle can be used for a perpendicular injection. Usually, many doctors use a cannula and the author uses a relatively big diameter cannula such as 21G.

(Tip) Diameter of cannula (Table 3.3): There are a lot of controversies in which the cannula is better to use. But when smaller than 27G, a cannula is the same as a needle [6]. A bigger cannula can help prevent perforating the artery. So the author likes to use a 21G cannula.

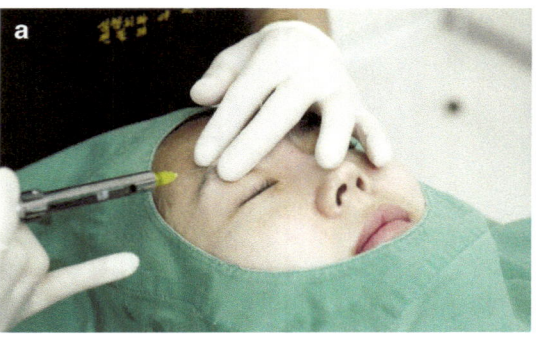 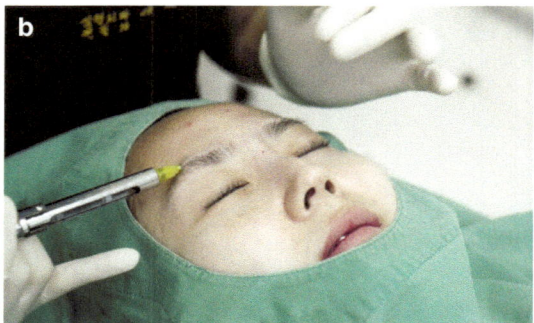

Fig. 3.5 (**a**) Entry point anesthesia and (**b**) Regional anesthesia at the supratrochlear nerve and supraorbital nerve

Table 3.3 Needle gauge outer diameter and inner diameter

Needle gauge	Outer diameter (mm)	Inner diameter (mm)
18	1.27	0.84
20	0.91	0.6
21	0.82	0.51
25	0.51	0.26
27	0.41	0.21
30	0.31	0.16

3.8 Entry Point

The lateral eyebrow is used as an entry point. When using a cannula, after the entry point is made, insert the cannula into the subgaleal plane and inject filler. When creating an entry point at the lateral portion of the hairline, a cannula cannot reach the central forehead. 2 cm above the eyebrow is a reasonable entry point considering the arterial pathway but the supraorbital artery has variation in how it runs so there is no 100% safe location of an entry point [7]. Another entry point might be at the hairline but it might be a dangerous technique for two reasons. One is the cannula is directed toward the eye and second is since the skull is curved, the cannula also should be curved and it is hard to locate the cannula tip at the subgaleal position [8].

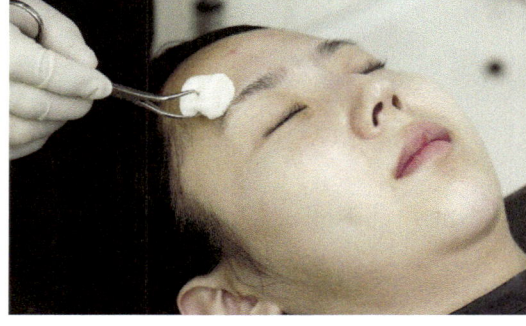

Fig. 3.6 Performing sterilization and anesthesia (Fig. 3.5)

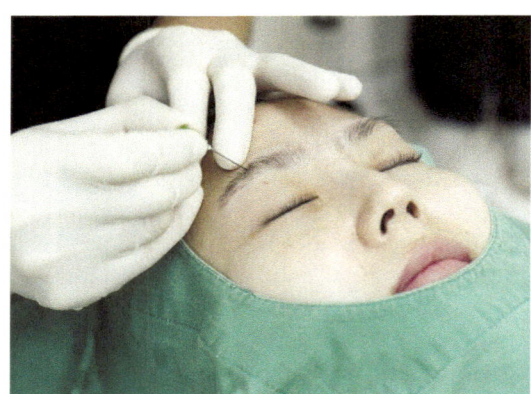

Fig. 3.7 Puncture for entry point

3.9 Procedures (Figs. 3.6, 3.7, 3.8, 3.9, 3.10, 3.11 and 3.12)

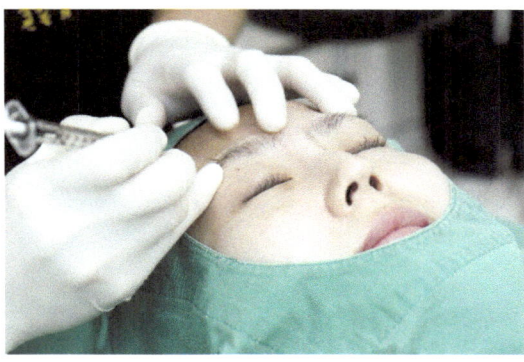

Fig. 3.8 Perforating frontalis muscle to enter subgaleal plane by cannula

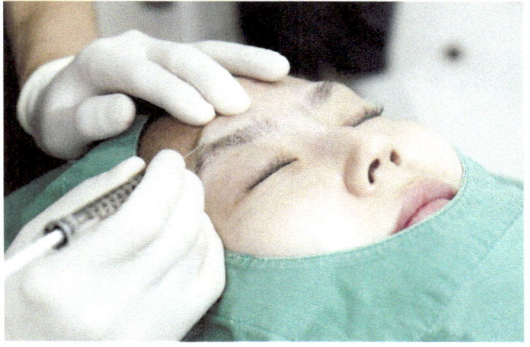

Fig. 3.9 Approach the cannula tip gently for the desired location of HA injection

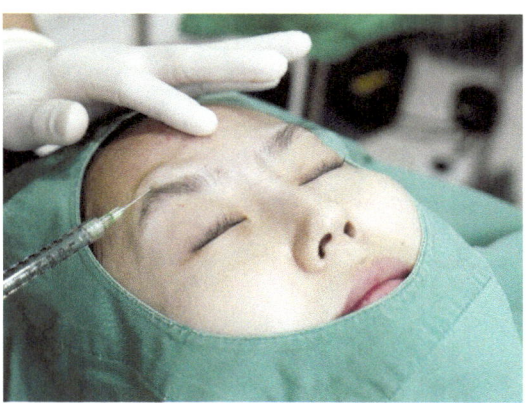

Fig. 3.10 Inject HA filler gently. Inject HA filler no more than 0.1 mL at one point

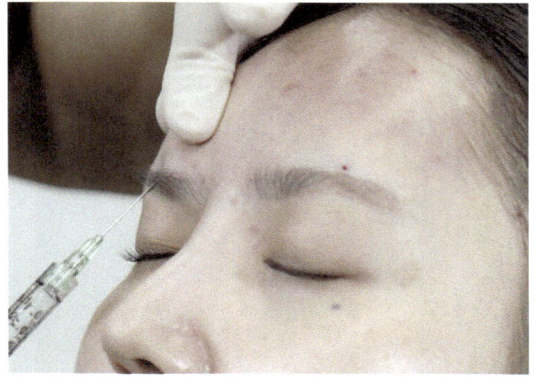

Fig. 3.11 Put patient in upright position and inject little by little for correction of irregularity

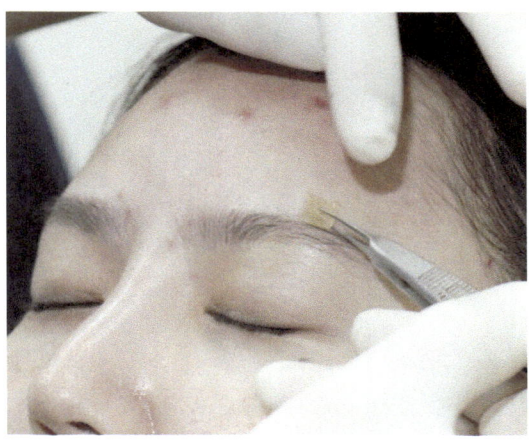

Fig. 3.12 Hydrocolloid applied

3.10   Pre and Postop Photograph
(Figs. 3.13 and 3.14)

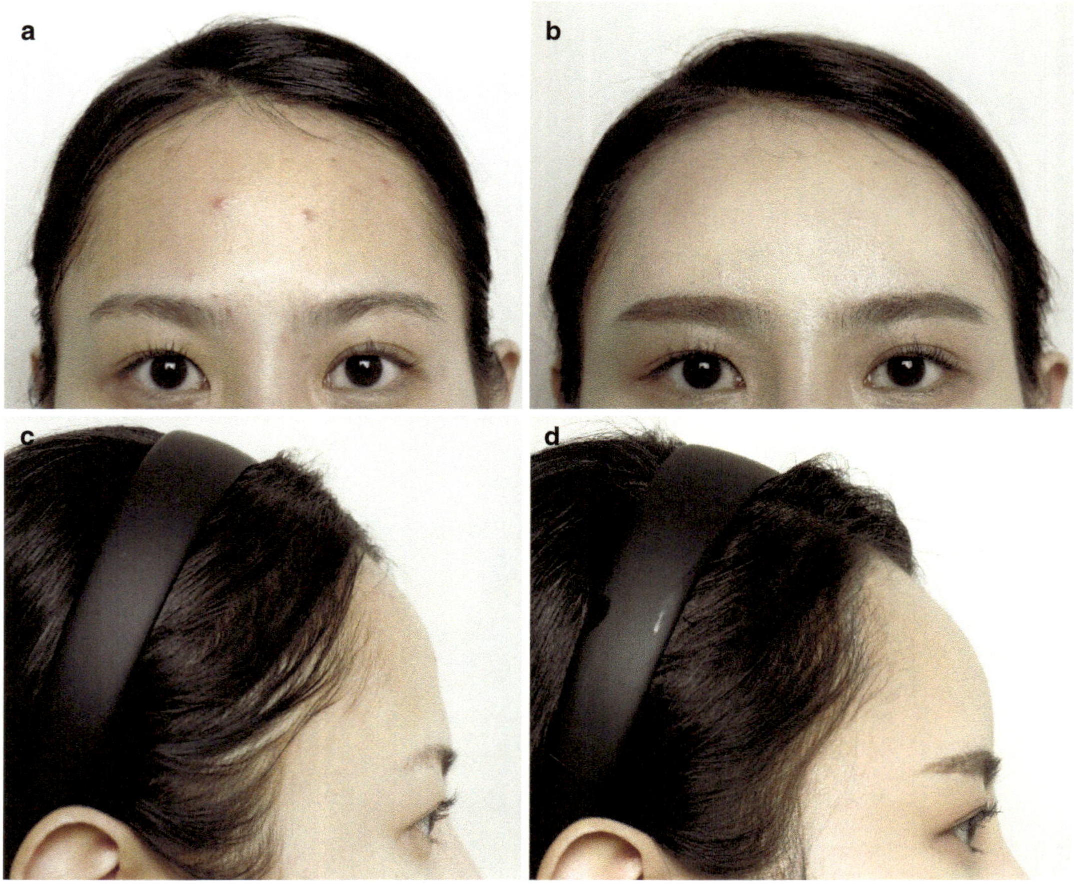

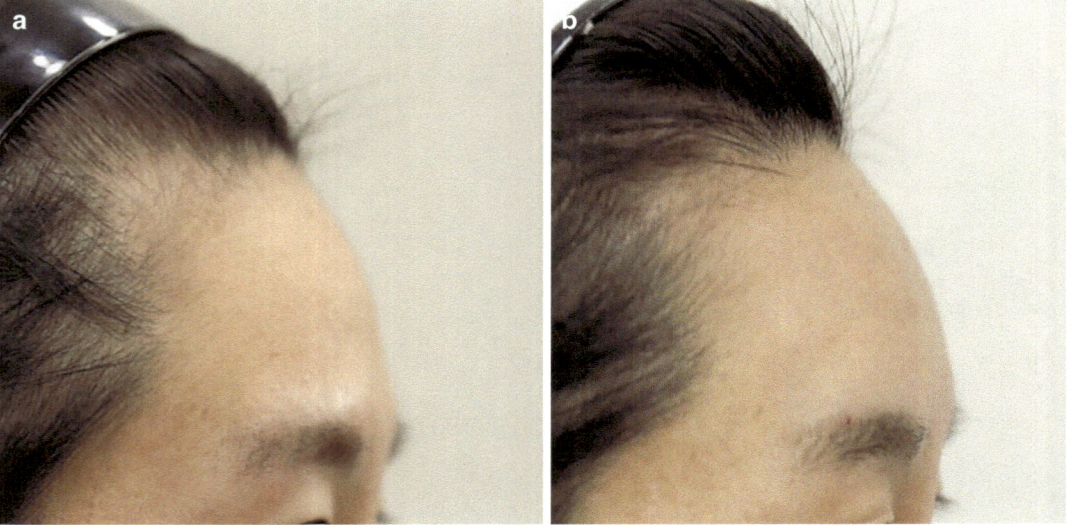

Fig. 3.13 A 23-year-old female patient, Forehead HA filler 3 mL. (**a**) Preop frontal view, (**b**) Postop 2 week frontal view, (**c**) Preop lateral view, and (**d**) Postop 2 week lateral view

Fig. 3.14 A 28-year-old female patient, Forehead HA filler 3 mL. (**a**) Preop lateral view and (**b**) Postop lateral view

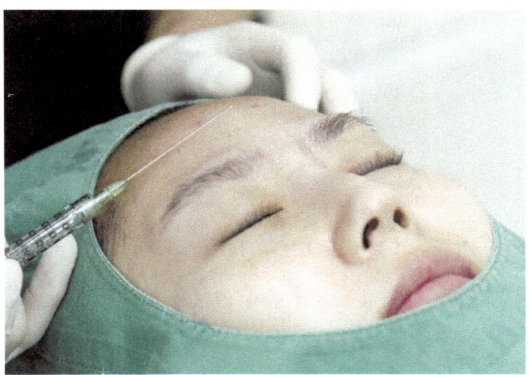

Fig. 3.15 Making entry point at lateral portion of forehead using cannula

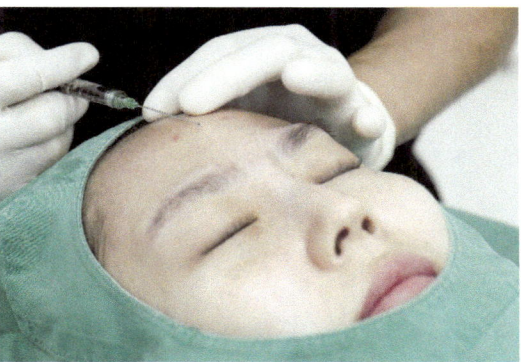

Fig. 3.16 Making entry point at the hairline using cannula

3.11   Other Techniques

3.11.1   Make an Entry Point in the Lateral Portion of the Forehead Using a Cannula (Fig. 3.15)

Anatomically, the supraorbital artery tends to perforate the frontalis muscle 2 cm above the eyebrow, so it is reasonable to make the entry point 2 cm above the eyebrow and inject filler at the supraperiosteal layer. But the supraorbital artery's deep branch can reach 4 cm above the eyebrow and the supratrochlear artery could run a deep branch and superficial branch. These variations might occur, so there is no 100% safe technique. Also, there might be a risk of scarring because the cannula should move anterograde and retrograde and could possibly make a maceration scar [9]. The author personally does not perform this entry point.

3.11.2   Make the Entry Point at the Hairline and Use a Cannula (Fig. 3.16)

The entry point can be obscure but it is difficult to locate the cannula tip under the frontalis muscle when performing just above the supraorbital

ridge because the skull tends to be curved. Also, there are risks in meeting the supratrochlear artery and/or supraorbital artery because the direction is exactly opposite [10]. Also when creating a midline entry point, the central artery, which is a branch of the supratrochlear artery, can be perforated.

3.11.3   Botulinum Toxin Injection (Fig. 3.17)

For some patients who use their frontalis muscle often, it is recommended to inject botulinum toxin concomitantly because of prevention of filler migration.

> **Key**
> 1. High cohesiveness.
> 2. Layer: Subgaleal plane.
> 3. Artery: Supratrochlear artery, supraorbital artery, superficial temporal artery pathway.
> 4. Irregularity is a common complication of forehead HA filler injection. So the subgaleal layer and molding are important.
> 5. Not to inject near the supraorbital ridge.

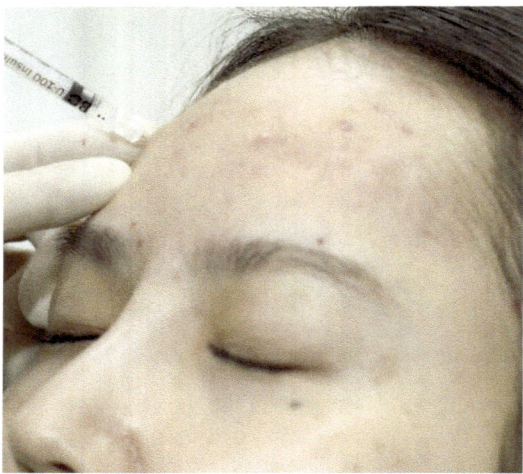

Fig. 3.17 Forehead botulinum toxin injection

References

1. Cotofana S, Mian A, Sykes JM, Redka-Swoboda W, Ladinger A, Pavicic T, Schenck TL, Benslimane F, Ingallina F, Schlattau A. An update on the anatomy of the forehead compartments. Plast Reconstr Surg. 2017 Apr;139(4):864e–872e. https://doi.org/10.1097/PRS.0000000000003174.

2. Tansatit T, Phumyoo T, Jitaree B, Sawatwong W, Rungsawang C, Jiirasutat N, Sahraoui YME, Lee JH. Ultrasound evaluation of arterial anastomosis of the forehead. J Cosmet Dermatol. 2018 Dec;17(6):1031–6. https://doi.org/10.1111/jocd.12755.

3. van Loghem JAJ, Humzah D, Kerscher M. Cannula versus sharp needle for placement of soft tissue fillers: an observational cadaver study. Aesthet Surg J. 2017 Dec 13;38(1):73–88. https://doi.org/10.1093/asj/sjw220.

4. Pavicic T, Yankova M, Schenck TL, Frank K, Freytag DL, Sykes J, Green JB, Hamade H, Casabona G, Cotofana S. Subperiosteal injections during facial soft tissue filler injections-Is it possible? J Cosmet Dermatol. 2020 Mar;19(3):590–5. https://doi.org/10.1111/jocd.13073.

5. Rohrich RJ, Pessa JE. The fat compartments of the face: anatomy and clinical implications for cosmetic surgery. Plast Reconstr Surg. 2007 Jun;119(7):2219–27. https://doi.org/10.1097/01.prs.0000265403.66886.54.

6. Pavicic T, Webb KL, Frank K, Gotkin RH, Tamura B, Cotofana S. Arterial wall penetration forces in needles versus cannulas. Plast Reconstr Surg. 2019 Mar;143(3):504e–512e. https://doi.org/10.1097/PRS.0000000000005321.

7. Cong LY, Phothong W, Lee SH, Wanitphakdeedecha R, Koh I, Tansatit T, Kim HJ. Topographic analysis of the supratrochlear artery and the supraorbital artery: implication for improving the safety of forehead augmentation. Plast Reconstr Surg. 2017 Mar;139(3):620e–627e. https://doi.org/10.1097/PRS.0000000000003060.

8. Lee W. Prevention of hyaluronic acid filler-induced blindness. Dermatol Ther. 2020 Jul;33(4):e13657. https://doi.org/10.1111/dth.13657.

9. Kim J. Novel forehead augmentation strategy: forehead depression categorization and calcium-hydroxyapatite filler delivery after tumescent injection. Plast Reconstr Surg Glob Open. 2018 Sep 6;6(9):e1858. https://doi.org/10.1097/GOX.0000000000001858.

10. Tansatit T, Apinuntrum P, Phetudom T. A dark side of the cannula injections: how arterial wall perforations and emboli occur. Aesthet Plast Surg. 2017 Feb;41(1):221–7. https://doi.org/10.1007/s00266-016-0725-7.

Glabellar wrinkle lines appear differently depending on individual patients, but usually show vertical lines medial from the eyebrow. Wrinkles develop because of repetitive contraction of the corrugator supercilii muscle and procerus muscle. So botulinum toxin must be injected to correct glabellar wrinkle lines. When a wrinkle shows even if botulinum toxin is injected, hyaluronic acid filler injection should be considered. HA injection always has the risk of vascular complications and is also applied at the glabellar wrinkle line. The glabellar is one of the danger zones for HA filler injection [1].

4.1 Vascular Anatomy

Glabellar wrinkle lines are often located where the supratrochlear artery pathway is (Fig. 4.1). Glabellar wrinkle lines develop because of the thin dermal of the subcutaneous layer, so a filler injection should be at the dermal layer or upper subcutaneous layer. When performing glabellar wrinkle correction, a detour of the supratrochlear artery is needed.

4.2 Injection Layer

The mechanism of glabellar wrinkle lines is repetitive movement of muscle and in consequence, dermal and/or subcutaneous fat atrophy

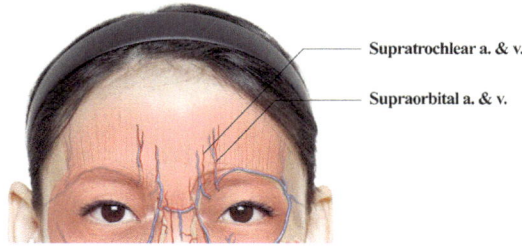

Fig. 4.1 Relationship between glabellar wrinkle line and supratrochlear artery

develops (Fig. 4.2). So when injecting HA filler, the target layer should be the dermal and/or subcutaneous layer. The most important thing is the pathway of the supratrochlear artery.

The supratrochlear artery runs too deep layers and perforates muscle usually at 2 cm above the eyebrow [2]. But variations also exist and the subdermal location can be detected by Doppler ultrasound [3]. When HA filler is injected into the supratrochlear artery, ocular complications could develop, so the glabellar area is one of the common causes of ocular complications [4].

4.3 Doppler Ultrasound Findings

The supratrochlear artery can be detected at the glabella area by doppler ultrasound. Avoiding injecting the artery is most important. The artery is located laterally from the glabellar

Fig. 4.2 Injection layer of glabellar wrinkle line. The injection layer should be the dermal layer or upper subcutaneous layer

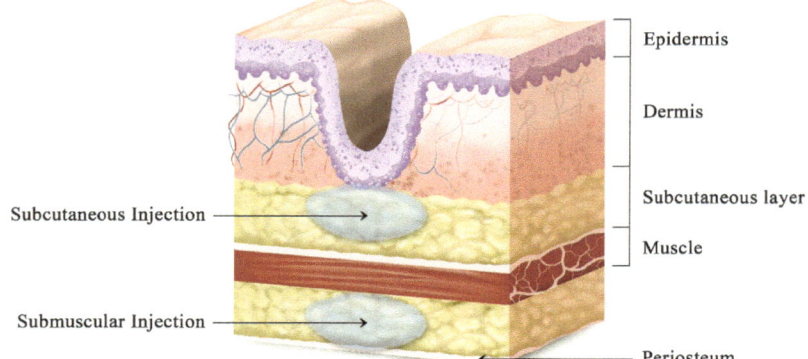

Fig. 4.3 The supratrochlear artery is located laterally from the glabellar wrinkle line

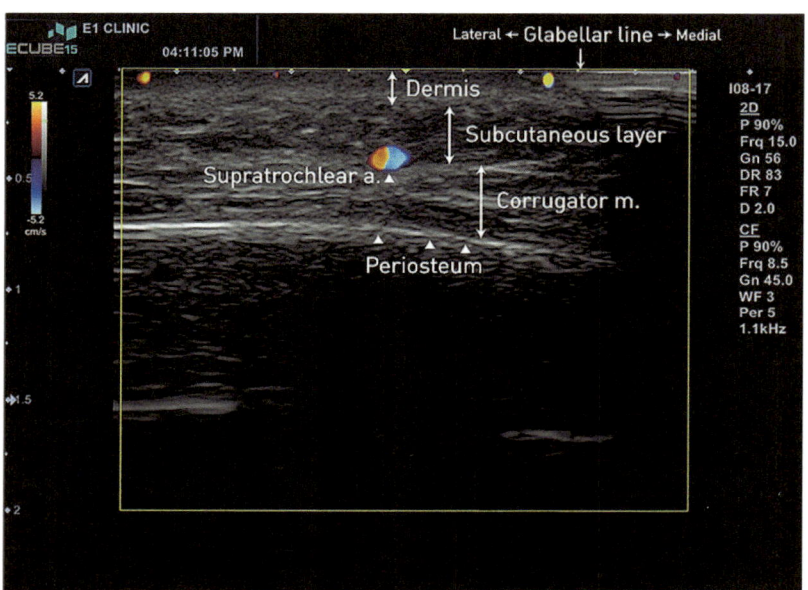

wrinkle line (Fig. 4.3) so filler can be injected under glabellar wrinkle lines. But when the artery is located at the line (Fig. 4.4) it is impossible to inject HA filler, so we recommend not to inject for a glabellar wrinkle correction.

4.4   Filler Choice

It is important to lift the skin for wrinkle correction but since the injection is performed at the dermal and/or subdermal layer, the filler should not be too hard (Table 4.1).

Fig. 4.4 The supratrochlear artery is located at the glabellar wrinkle line. When performing filler injection procedure, arterial penetration can occur

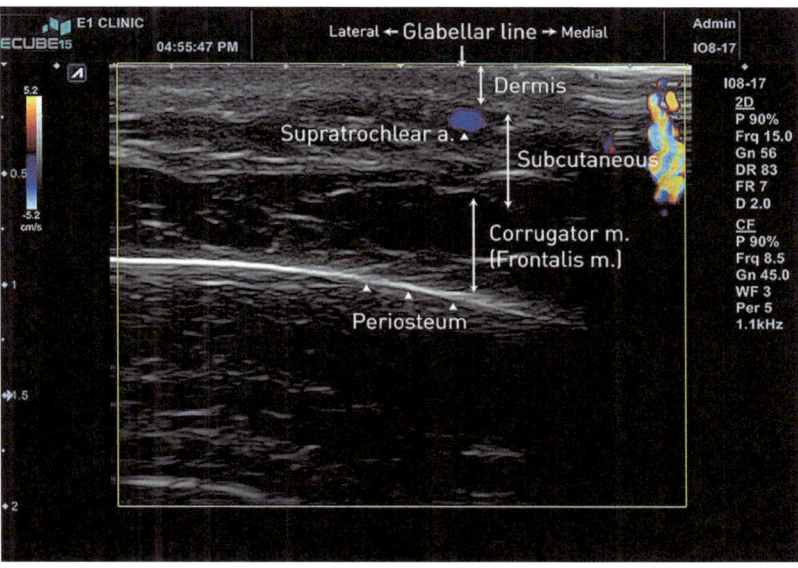

Table 4.1 Lorient rheologic test results

Product	G′ (Pa)	G″ (Pa)	Complex viscosity (μ)	Tan delta	Cohesiveness (N)
Lorient No. 2	203	41	1,673,007	0.20	0.4401
Lorient No. 4	338	95	2,795,776	0.28	0.4237
Lorient No. 6	413	121	3,423,232	0.29	0.4454

The author uses No. 2 or No. 4 for glabellar wrinkle line correction

4.5   Anesthesia

Localized anesthesia is needed so use topical anesthetic ointment.

4.6   Needle vs Cannula

A precise injection is needed for wrinkle correction so the author usually uses a needle after doppler ultrasound finding.

4.7   Injection Techniques
(Figs. 4.5, 4.6, 4.7, 4.8, and 4.9)

Glabellar wrinkle filler injection is a very simple method but the author always uses the Doppler ultrasound before correction. The most important thing is to prevent vascular complications. It is always recommended to use botulinum toxin.

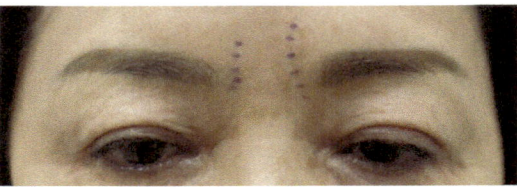

Fig. 4.5 Design the correction of glabellar wrinkle lines

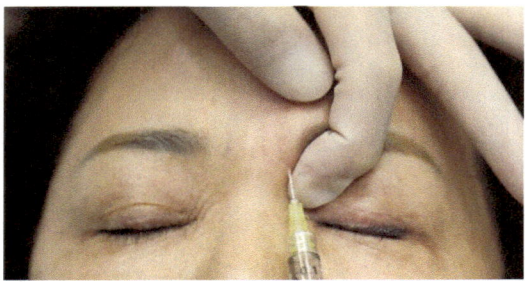

Fig. 4.8 Inject HA filler. Use 27G ~ 30G needle and direct needle far from the eye. It is recommended to compress the medial side of the orbit

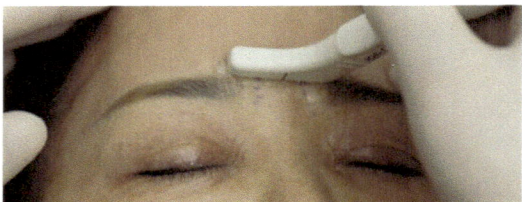

Fig. 4.6 Detect supratrochlear artery by doppler ultrasound

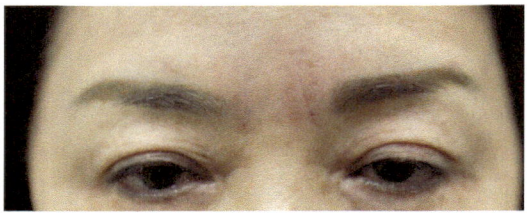

Fig. 4.9 Immediately after HA filler injection

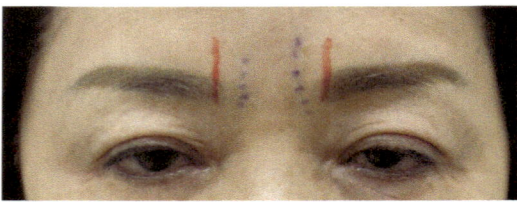

Fig. 4.7 Draw the detected artery

References

1. Scheuer JF 3rd, Sieber DA, Pezeshk RA, Gassman AA, Campbell CF, Rohrich RJ. Facial danger zones: techniques to maximize safety during soft-tissue filler injections. Plast Reconstr Surg. 2017 May;139(5):1103–8. https://doi.org/10.1097/PRS.0000000000003309.
2. Cong LY, Phothong W, Lee SH, Wanitphakdeedecha R, Koh I, Tansatit T, Kim HJ. Topographic analysis of the supratrochlear artery and the supraorbital artery: implication for improving the safety of forehead augmentation. Plast Reconstr Surg. 2017 Mar;139(3):620e–7e. https://doi.org/10.1097/PRS.0000000000003060.
3. Lee W, Moon HJ, Kim JS, Yang EJ. Safe glabellar wrinkle correction with soft tissue filler using doppler ultrasound. Aesthet Surg J. 2020 Jul 9:sjaa197. https://doi.org/10.1093/asj/sjaa197.
4. Beleznay K, Carruthers JD, Humphrey S, Jones D. Avoiding and treating blindness from fillers: a review of the world literature. Dermatol Surg. 2015 Oct;41(10):1097–117. https://doi.org/10.1097/DSS.0000000000000486.

5.1   Anatomy and Considerations

The temple area is composed of the skull including the frontal bone, parietal bone, temporal bone, and sphenoid bone and is covered by multiple thick soft tissues. The temple is defined from the superior temporal septum to the zygomatic arch. For Oriental patients, a prominent zygomatic arch is common, so relatively depressed temple areas are found. Augmenting the temple area can make a natural curvature from the forehead to zygoma line.

From the outer surface, the temple area is composed of complex layers including skin, subcutaneous layer, superficial temporal fascia, deep temporal fascia, temporalis muscle, and bone (Fig. 5.1). There is also loose areolar tissue between the STF and DTF and innominate fascia, parotid temporal fascia can be found depends on the height of the temple area [1].

There are three possible layers to inject hyaluronic acid filler. First, a superficial injection that is injected at the subcutaneous layer, second is to inject between the STF and DTF, and third is a deep injection which is to inject under the temporalis muscle by touching the bone by needle end [2]. There is a fat layer between the temporalis muscle and DTF but this is the temporal extension of the buccal fat pad, so injecting into this layer can cause filler migration to the buccal area. The easiest technique is to inject deeply by touching the bone with the needle end. But recently

multiple problems have been found with this technique. First, a case was reported of penetration of the temporal bone [3]. Deep temporal fascia is very hard tissue so it is hard to perforate it with a cannula. But a needle can penetrate both the DTF and temporal muscle and the temporal bone has a very thin structure and there is possibility of destruction. Second, the temporalis muscle is part of the mastication muscle and a periosteum does not exist. Thus, the temporalis muscle is stuck very firmly to the bone and injecting deeply means to inject into the temporalis muscle rather than the supraperiosteal layer [4]. Continuous shearing forces are applied because of temporalis muscle action by mastication. Other possible problems of deep injection are given in Table 5.1.

The author likes to inject between the STF and DTF because the superficial temporal artery and temporal branch of the facial nerve like to run shielded by the STF and a cannula can puncture the STF easily, so a relatively safe plane is exposed. Compared to a deep injection, a small amount of HA filler can show better results.

The important vessels at the temple area are the superficial temporal artery, sentinel vein, middle temporal vein, and deep temporal artery. When performing palpation to the temple area, the superficial temporal artery tends to pulsate (Fig. 5.2) [7]. The superficial temporal artery is a branch of the external carotid artery and runs vertically anterior from the ear. The frontal branch of

Fig. 5.1 Multiple layers of temple area

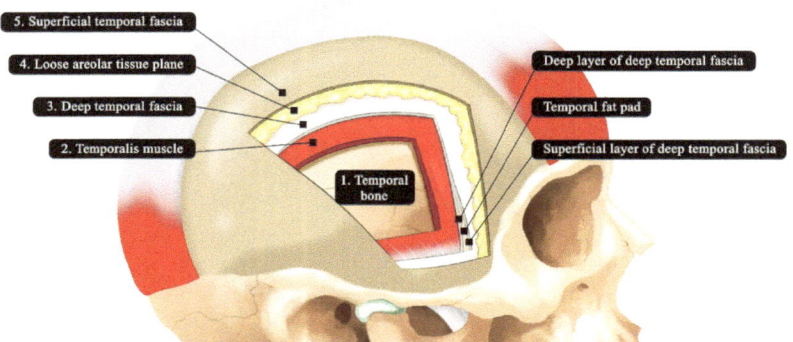

Table 5.1 Disadvantages of deep injection of temple area

1. Case report of penetrating temporal bone by needle [3].
2. The needle should be used for deep injection so there is possibility of vascular injury such as to the superficial temporal artery, anterior branch of deep temporal artery, or middle temporal vein [5].
3. A relatively large amount of filler is needed.
4. Impossible to inject into the submuscular layer so longevity is decreased due to muscle action [4].
5. Difficult to eliminate when granuloma occurs [6].

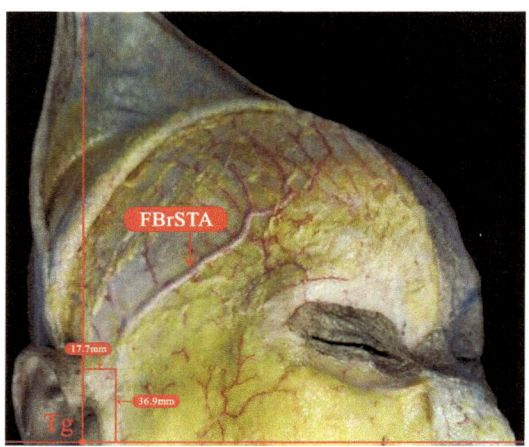

Fig. 5.2 Cadaveric finding of superficial temporal artery

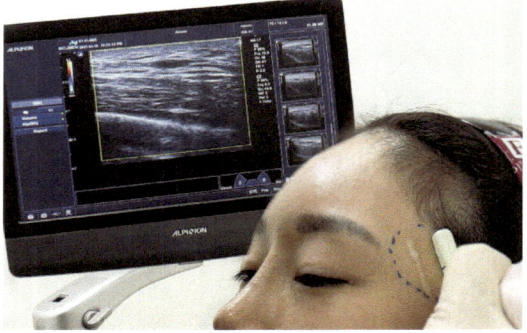

Fig. 5.3 Ultrasound detection of temple area

the STA runs superficially at the temple area. The STA is a relatively large vessel so it is easily detected by Doppler ultrasound (Fig. 5.3).

A guide is proposed of a perpendicular injection at the site of 1 cm upper and 1 cm lateral from the eyebrow end [8], however, this technique has the risk of perforating the superficial temporal artery, zygomatico-orbital artery, and anterior branch of the deep temporal artery. In ultrasound scans, both arteries, the STA and the DTA, can be detected (Fig. 5.4). This area is also close to the area known as the zone of caution, which is the area where the sentinel vein perforates superficially and there is a superficial perforation of the temporal branch of the facial nerve [9]. A deep perpendicular injection is the easiest technique but doctors should be careful with the relationship between the arteries of the temple (Fig. 5.5).

The middle temporal vein tends to run in the deep temporal fascia layer and 1 cm above the zygomatic arch level and runs deeply at the deep temporal fascia so an injection at the space between the STF and DTF is a safe location not interrupting the middle temporal vein [10].

The sentinel vein, known as the medial zygomatico temporal vein, is often visible at the lateral side of the forehead and is not at high risk until injected by a needle. But when a high amount of filler is injected into the temple area, this prominent vein can be shown. So when this vein is visible before an injection, making the patient perform the Valsalva maneuver could assist in estimating the result. Preoperative informed consent is needed for prominent veins.

5.2 Filler Choice

The temple area is also a wide area so doctors should consider cohesiveness and given the final purpose is to lift, lifting capacity should also be considered. The author uses the layer between the STF and DTF so uses No. 4 at the temple area (Table 5.2).

5.3 Entry Point

When injection is performed by cannula, the entry points are at the hairline or near the eyebrow (Fig. 5.6).

5.4 Anesthesia

Usually a regional block (auriculotemporal nerve and/or zygomaticotemporal nerve block) is not performed. Usually local anesthesia is performed, injecting at the entry point and under the STF layer.

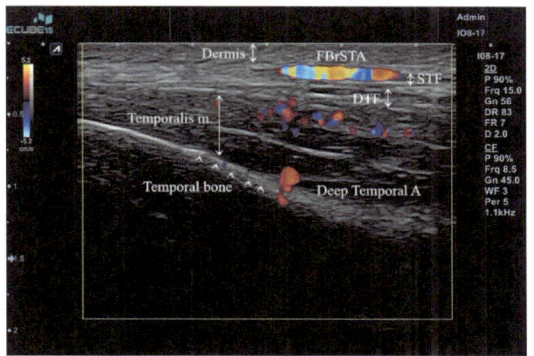

Fig. 5.4 Arteries of temple area by Doppler ultrasound (FBrSTA: Frontal branch of Superficial temporal artery and Deep temporal artery anterior branch)

Fig. 5.5 Arteries of temple area and what might be encountered by perpendicular deep injection

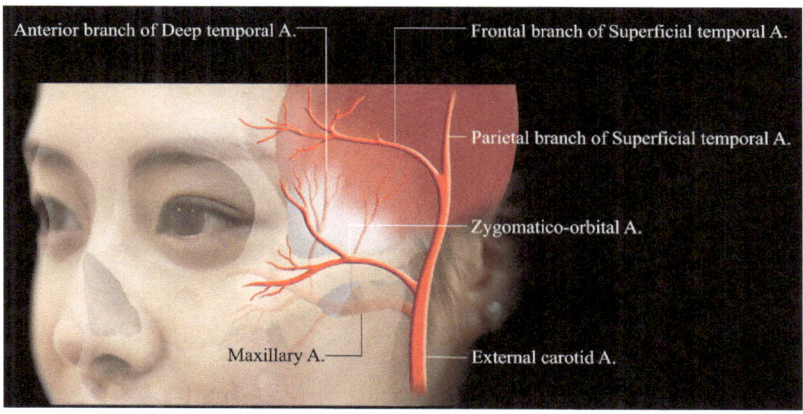

Table 5.2 Rheological results of Lorient HA filler

Product	G′ (Pa)	G″ (Pa)	Complex viscosity (μ)	Tan delta	Cohesiveness (N)
Lorient No. 2	203	41	1,673,007	0.20	0.4401
Lorient No. 4	338	95	2,795,776	0.28	0.4237
Lorient No. 6	413	121	3,423,232	0.29	0.4454

The author uses No. 4 for temple augmentation

5.5   Injection Techniques
(Figs. 5.7, 5.8, 5.9, 5.10, and 5.11)

Doppler ultrasound detection of the superficial temporal artery is performed. Then a local anesthesia is injected at the hairline. After a needle puncture of the entry point, a 21G cannula is inserted. The STF is perforated easily by cannula but the DTF is hard to perforate so the cannula tip can be located between the STF and DTF easily. Inject HA filler when the cannula tip is located correctly. Inject gently using the retrograde threading technique.

The superficial temporal artery is located at the STF so locate the cannula hole downward. The left hand can feel during HA filler injection.

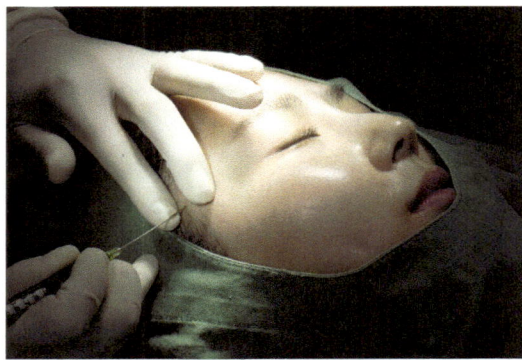

Fig. 5.8 Proceed gently with cannula tip between STF and DTF

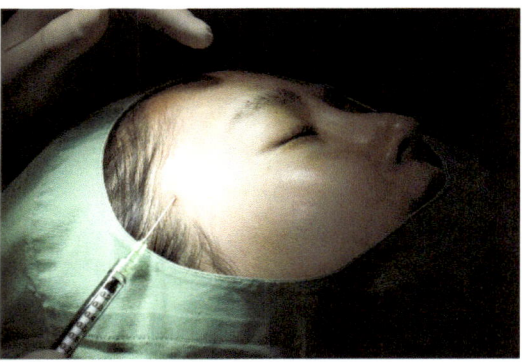

Fig. 5.9 Gentle injection by linear threading technique

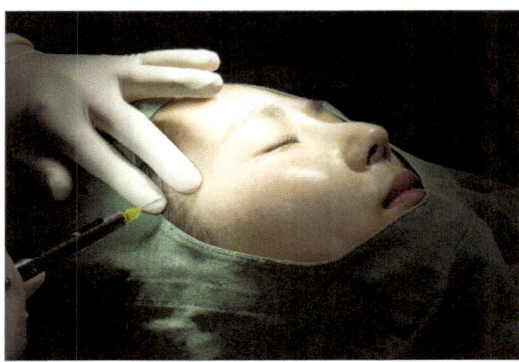

Fig. 5.6 Local anesthesia at entry point

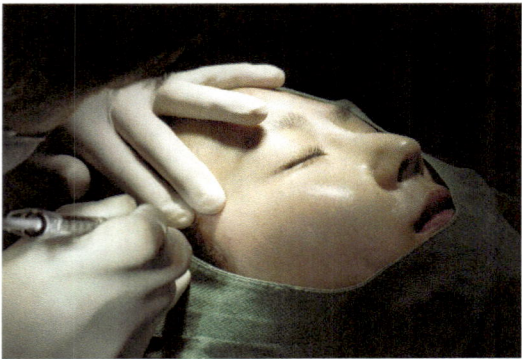

Fig. 5.7 Approach 21G cannula between STF and DTF. STF is easily perforated

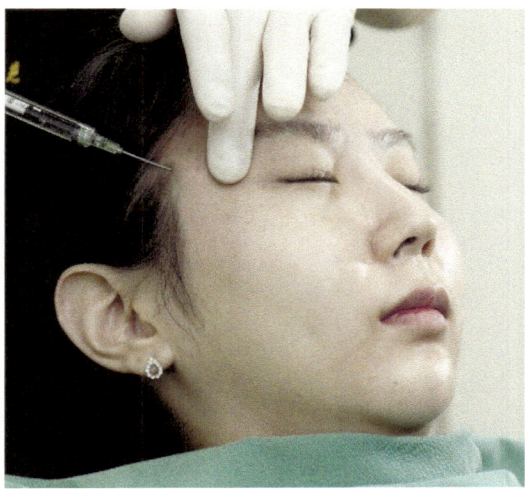

Fig. 5.10 Place the patient in upright position and inject filler if there is insufficient location

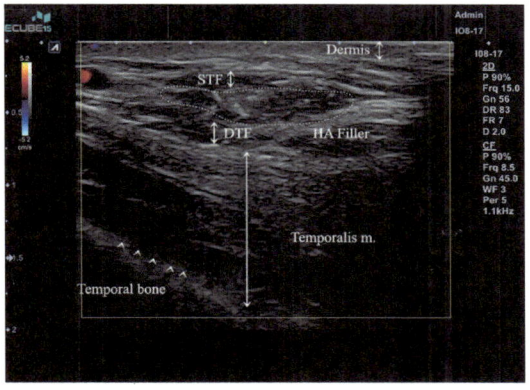

Fig. 5.11 Ultrasound finding after HA filler injection. (HA filler: dotted)

5.6   Pre- and Post-procedural Photograph (Figs. 5.12 and 5.13)

Key

1. Layer: Between superficial temporal fascia and deep temporal fascia, subcutaneous layer.
2. Vessels: Superficial temporal artery, sentinel vein, middle temporal vein, and anterior branch of deep temporal artery.

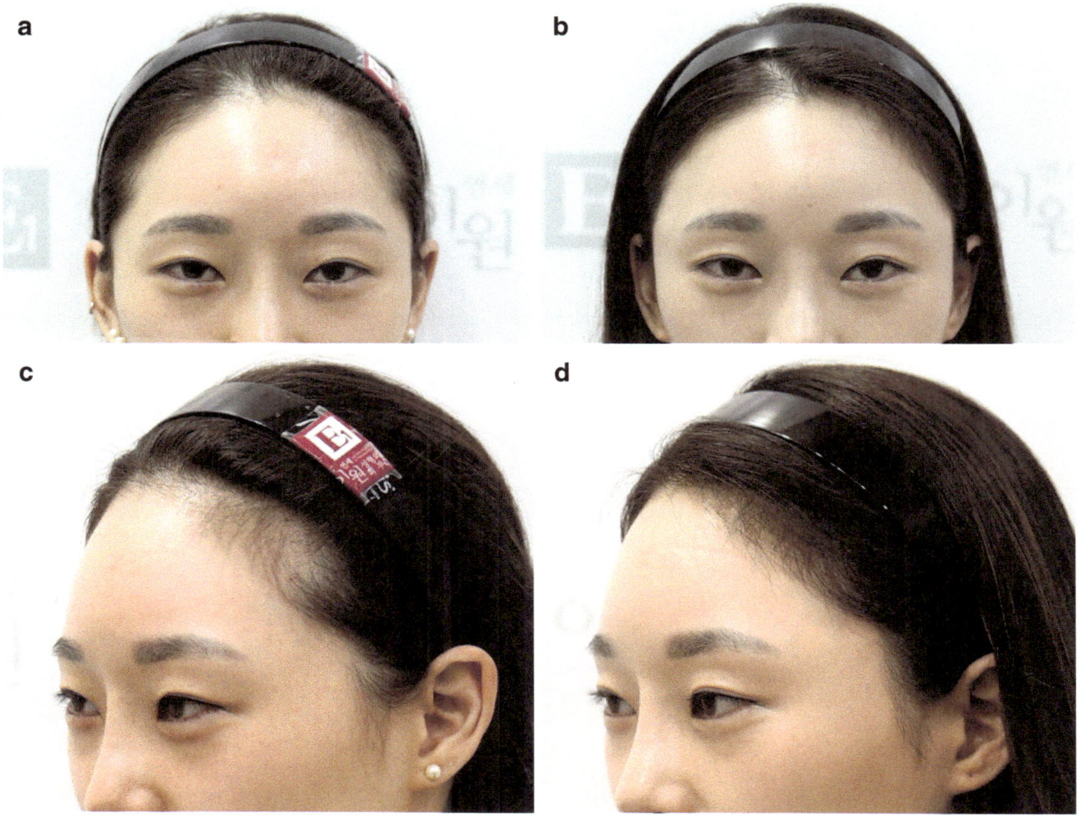

Fig. 5.12 A 29-year-old patient. 0.8 mL of HA filler is injected bilaterally. (**a**) Pre-procedural front view, (**b**) Post 3 month front view, (**c**) Pre-procedural three-quarter view, and (**d**) Post 3 month three quarter view

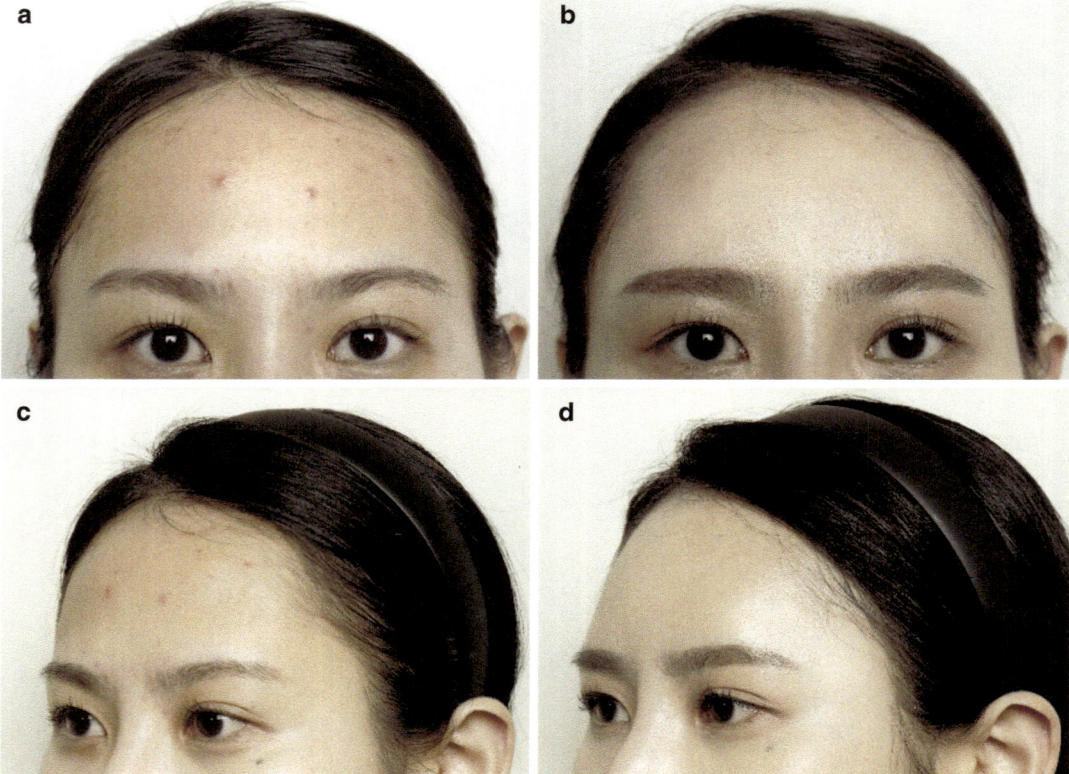

Fig. 5.13 A 23-year-old patient. 1 mL of HA filler is injected bilaterally. (**a**) Pre-procedural front view, (**b**) Post 2 week front view, (**c**) Pre-procedural three-quarter view, and (**d**) Post 2 week three-quarter view

References

1. Davidge KM, van Furth WR, Agur A, Cusimano M. Naming the soft tissue layers of the temporoparietal region: unifying anatomic terminology across surgical disciplines. Neurosurgery. 2010 Sep;67(3 Suppl Operative):ons120–9.
2. Breithaupt AD, Jones DH, Braz A, Narins R, Weinkle S. Anatomical basis for safe and effective volumization of the temple. Dermatol Surg. 2015 Dec;41(Suppl 1):S278–83. https://doi.org/10.1097/DSS.0000000000000539.
3. Philipp-Dormston WG, Bieler L, Hessenberger M, Schenck TL, Frank K, Fierlbeck J, et al. Intracranial penetration during temporal soft tissue filler injection-is it possible? Dermatol Surg. 2018;44(1):84–91.
4. van Loghem JAJ, Humzah D, Kerscher M. Cannula versus sharp needle for placement of soft tissue fillers: an observational cadaver study. Aesthet Surg J. 2017 Dec 13;38(1):73–88. https://doi.org/10.1093/asj/sjw220.
5. Carruthers J, Humphrey S, Beleznay K, Carruthers A. Suggested injection zone for soft tissue fillers in the temple? Dermatol Surg. 2017;43(5):756–7.
6. Lee JM, Kim YJ. Foreign body granulomas after the use of dermal fillers: pathophysiology, clinical appearance, histologic features, and treatment. Arch Plast Surg. 2015;42(2):232–9.
7. Lee J-G, Yang H-M, Hu K-S, et al. Frontal branch of the superficial temporal artery: anatomical study and clinical implications regarding injectable treatments. Surg Radiol Anat. 2015;37(1):61–8.
8. Sykes JM, Cotofana S, Trevidic P, Solish N, Carruthers J, Carruthers A, et al. Upper face: clinical anatomy and regional approaches with injectable fillers. Plast Reconstr Surg. 2015;136(5 Suppl):204s–18s.
9. Trinei FA, Januszkiewicz J, Nahai F. The sentinel vein: an important reference point for surgery in the temporal region. Plast Reconstr Surg. 1998 Jan;101(1):27–32. https://doi.org/10.1097/00006534-199801000-00006.
10. Jung W, Youn KH, Won SY, Park JT, Hu KS, Kim HJ. Clinical implications of the middle temporal vein with regard to temporal fossa augmentation. Dermatol Surg. 2014;40(6):618–23.

In the aspect of the nose, there is little difference between Oriental patients and Western patients. Western patients usually have a high dorsum of the nose so HA filler is used for some depressed areas or for correction of deviations. So, a small amount of needle is usually performed [1]. For Oriental patients, HA injections are performed because of the low dorsum [2]. So, a relatively large amount of filler is injected and the vascular anatomy is extremely important. The nose can be divided into the radix, rhinion, supratip, and tip area and it is important to know the vascular anatomy and layers of each injected area [3].

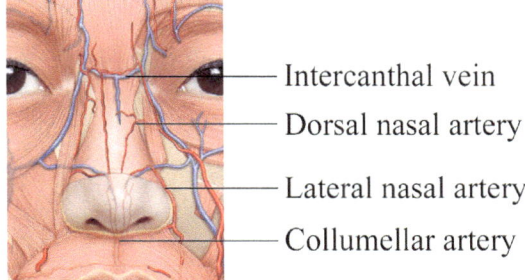

Fig. 6.1 Vascular anatomy of the nose

6.1 Radix and Rhinion

6.1.1 Anatomy and General Considerations

One of the most common filler procedures can be to augment the dorsum of the nose. There are two possible layers for filler injection and those are the subdermal layer and supraperiosteal layer. In cadaveric studies, the arteries and veins are running above the fibromuscular layer so injecting at the supraperiosteal layer is known for being a safe injection plane [4]. But when applying the Doppler ultrasound, some dorsal nasal arterial branches are detected at the supraperiosteal layer so there are no 100% safe places for injection [2].

We can estimate that the pressure of nose arteries is not high because the branch of the external carotid artery (ophthalmic artery) and branch of the internal carotid artery (facial artery) anastomosis at the nose (Fig. 6.1). Thus, when performing filler injection, low injection pressure might affect the ophthalmic artery. A previous article described that the glabellar area is the most common area for ocular complications [5]. But an updated article described that an injection at the nose is the most common area of ocular complications [6]. Thus, doctors should be aware that the injection rhinoplasty is a very dangerous procedure.

6.1.2 Doppler Ultrasound Findings

We can detect the arterial pathway before filler injection at the nose. A probe should be attached at the nose to detect vascular anatomy (Figs. 6.2 and 6.3).

6.1.3 Injection Technique

Many doctors prefer to inject using an infralobule approach with a cannula [4]. The cannula should be located at the supraperiosteal layer. But this technique can cause vascular injury when the

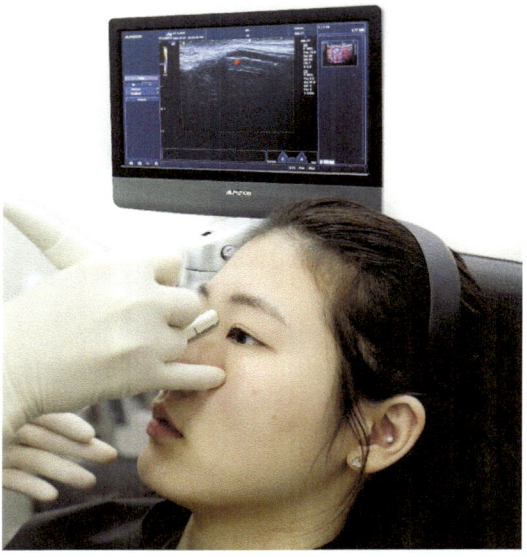

Fig. 6.2 Doppler ultrasound finding of the nose

cannula tip is tilted a little to approach the subcutaneous layer. For example, in nose hump cases, the cannula tip is likely to be located at the subcutaneous layer after passing the hump area and has a risk of vascular injury. When performing a perpendicular injection, the needle tip can be located at the supraperiosteal layer but the needle can encounter an artery and/or vein while approaching the layer [7]. Our study showed that if performing a perpendicular injection at the radix area, even if we performed a bone touch, the filler can be inserted into the dorsal nasal artery depending on the needle bevel location [8].

6.1.3.1 Infralobular Approach Technique by Cannula (Figs. 6.4, 6.5, 6.6, and 6.7)

6.1.3.2 Perpendicular Needle Injection (Figs. 6.8 and 6.9)

The nose injection is a common procedure in Oriental settings but is where vascular accidents most commonly occur. So it is most important to inject gently. Usually, the ejection pressure is higher than blood pressure so it is very important to inject slowly [9].

6.1.4 Widening Nose

Another consideration should be the hardness of filler. A few patients experience a widening of the injected nose as time goes by. This is because of the injected filler property and layer of injection. As described previously, a deep injection under

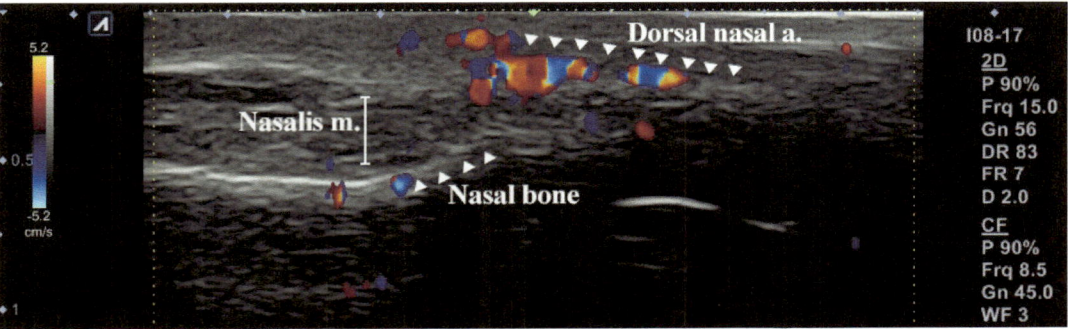

Fig. 6.3 Doppler ultrasound finding. Dorsal nasal artery can be detected just above the nasalis muscle

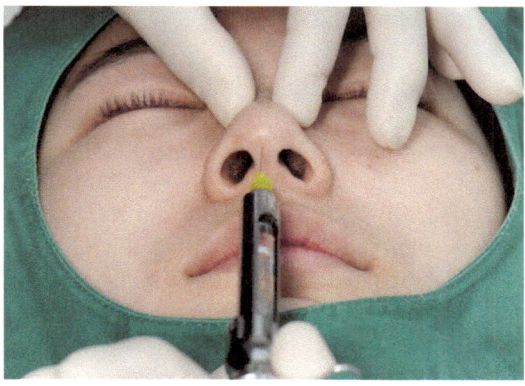

Fig. 6.4 Local lidocaine anesthesia at infralobular area

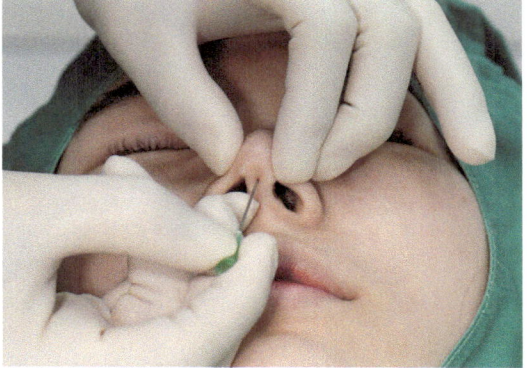

Fig. 6.5 Puncture by 21G needle

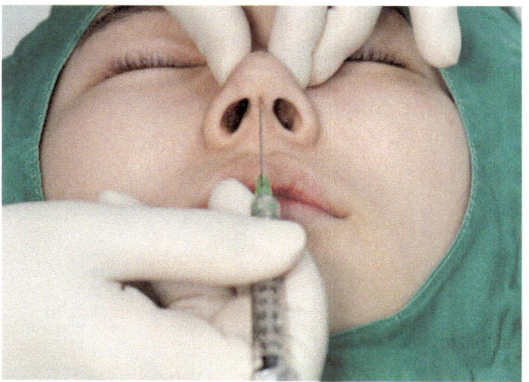

Fig. 6.6 Approach cannula tip

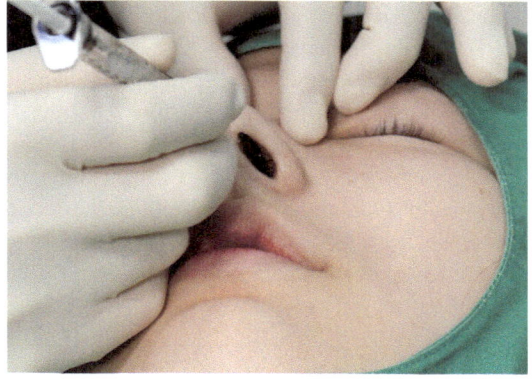

Fig. 6.7 When the cannula tip passes the nasal bone, the doctor should feel bone scratch (periosteum) to locate the supraperiosteal layer

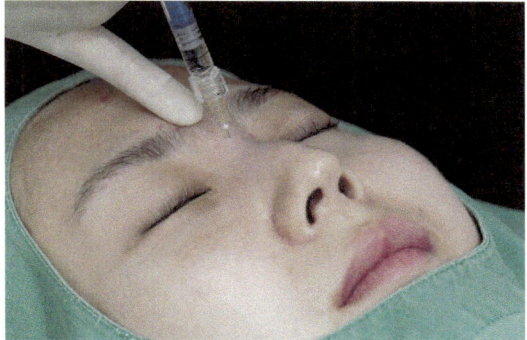

Fig. 6.8 Perpendicular needle injection. The needle tip should be located at the supraperiosteal layer (an aspiration test should be performed before the injection)

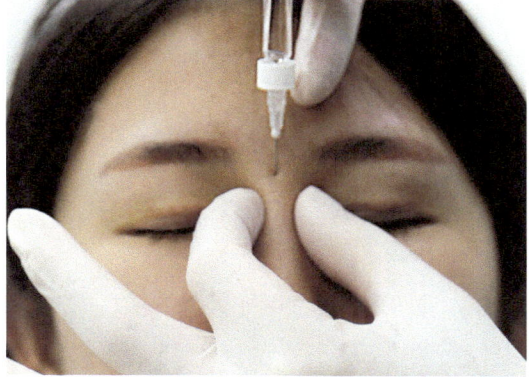

Fig. 6.9 When performing a nose injection, compression of the dorsal nasal artery pathway is recommended

muscle is a relatively safe place to inject, but the filler should be hard enough to resist the compression force by the nasalis muscle. When the injection is performed with a low G′ filler, it might spread to the lateral side. The author always uses a high G′ filler to inject under the muscle in such procedures as augmentation of the nose or chin. We can also consider a subdermal injection of a small amount of low G′ filler (Fig. 6.10).

6.1.5 Filler Choice

The author prefers high G′ biphasic filler. When performing a filler injection to the supraperiosteal layer, the filler should be hard enough to resist continuous compression force. So the author uses No. 6 for injections (Table 6.1).

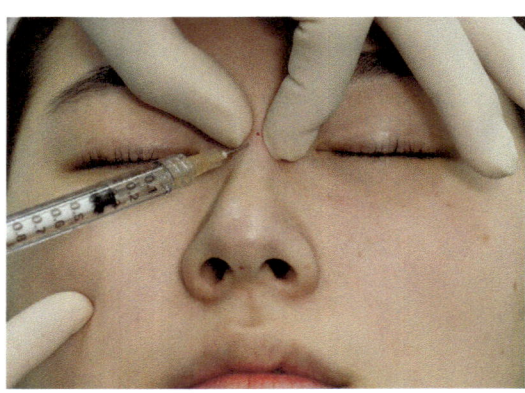

Fig. 6.10 Small amount of filler injection at subdermal layer

6.1.6 Needle Diameter

A lot of doctors use an insulin syringe or 30G needle for perpendicular injections [7]. But some HA fillers like to alter the property of the filler when passing a 30G needle. The author tested HA fillers by rheometer before and after passing the needle, and found out some fillers change their G' half parameter [10]. Usually, the 30G needle's inner diameter is 0.16 mm and when the filler's particle size is bigger, it might lose its own properties. So an appropriate choice of filler is needed.

> **Key**
> 1. Layer: Supraperiosteal layer, subdermal layer.
> 2. Filler: High G' filler when injecting at supraperiosteal layer.
> 3. Vessel: Dorsal nasal artery, lateral nasal artery, intercanthal vein.

6.2 Nasal Tip

The aesthetic profile combines the dorsum and tip of the nose. When performing operative rhinoplasty, an interdomal suture is essential for tip height. Recently tip augmentation using cogged threads has been used [11]. So when undertaking filler injection, tip augmentation is an essential procedure. But the problem is arterial supply. The dorsal nasal artery from ophthalmic artery, lateral nasal artery from facial artery, and columellar

Table 6.1 Rheologic Lorient results

Product	G′ (Pa)	G″ (Pa)	Complex viscosity (μ)	Tan delta	Cohesiveness (N)
Lorient No. 2	203	41	1,673,007	0.20	0.4401
Lorient No. 4	338	95	2,795,776	0.28	0.4237
Lorient No. 6	413	121	3,423,232	0.29	0.4454

The author uses No. 6 for nose augmentation

artery from superior labial artery all make anasto-mosis at the tip area. The nasal tip area consists of relatively thick skin and small diameter branches of arteries so there is a high risk of vascular complications, either an intravascular embolism or an extravascular compression. So a high amount of injection should be avoided (Fig. 6.11). Also, previous surgical rhinoplasty patients tend to ask for a tip plasty, but doctors should consider the destructed columellar artery resulting from the previous operation. So extreme caution is needed.

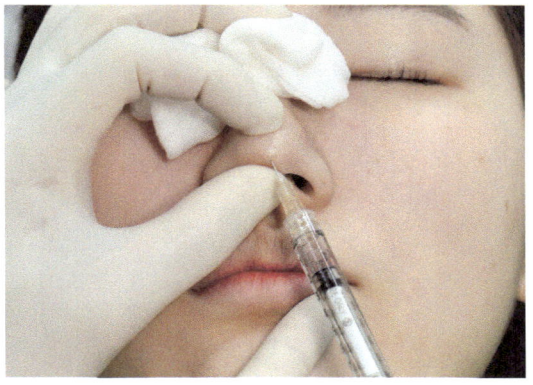

Fig. 6.11   Tip injection (0.1 mL by Lorient No. 2)

Key
1. Layer: Small amount of filler at near alar cartilage (0.1 ~ 0.2 mL).
2. Artery: Lateral nasal artery, dorsal nasal artery, columellar artery.

6.3   Pre- and Post-op Photograph of Nose Augmentation (Fig. 6.12)

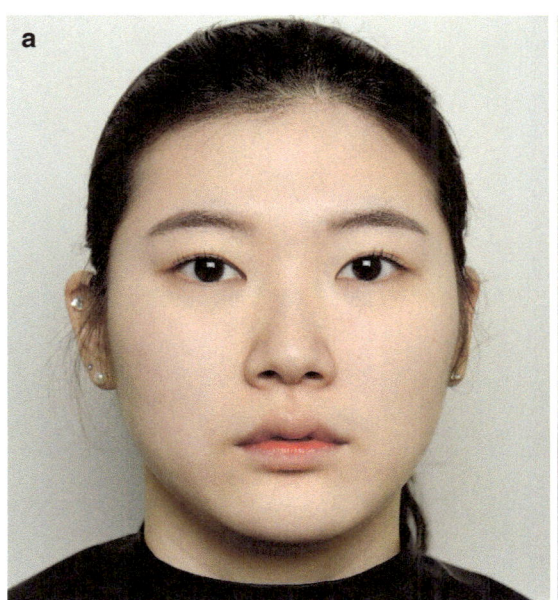
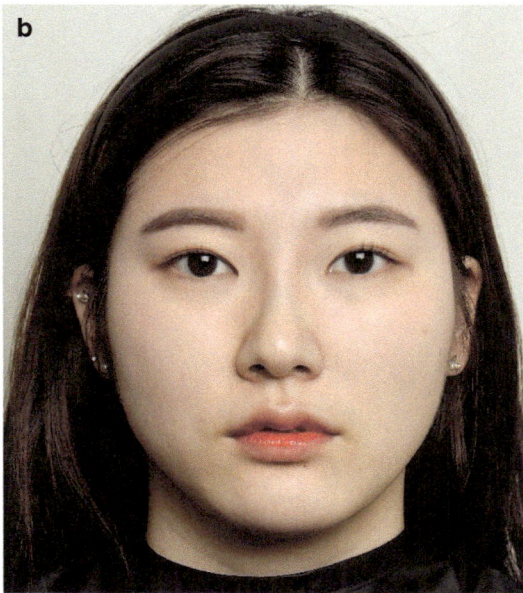

Fig. 6.12   Pre- and post-procedure photographs: Lorient No. 6 dorsum supraperiosteal layer 0.5 mL, Lorient No. 2 dorsum subdermal layer 0.1 mL, Lorient No. 2 tip 0.1 mL. (**a**) Pre-procedure front view, (**b**) Post-procedure 2 day front view, (**c**) Pre-procedure three-quarter view, (**d**) Post-procedure 2 day three-quarter view, (**e**) Pre-procedure lateral view, and (**f**) Post-procedure 2 day lateral view

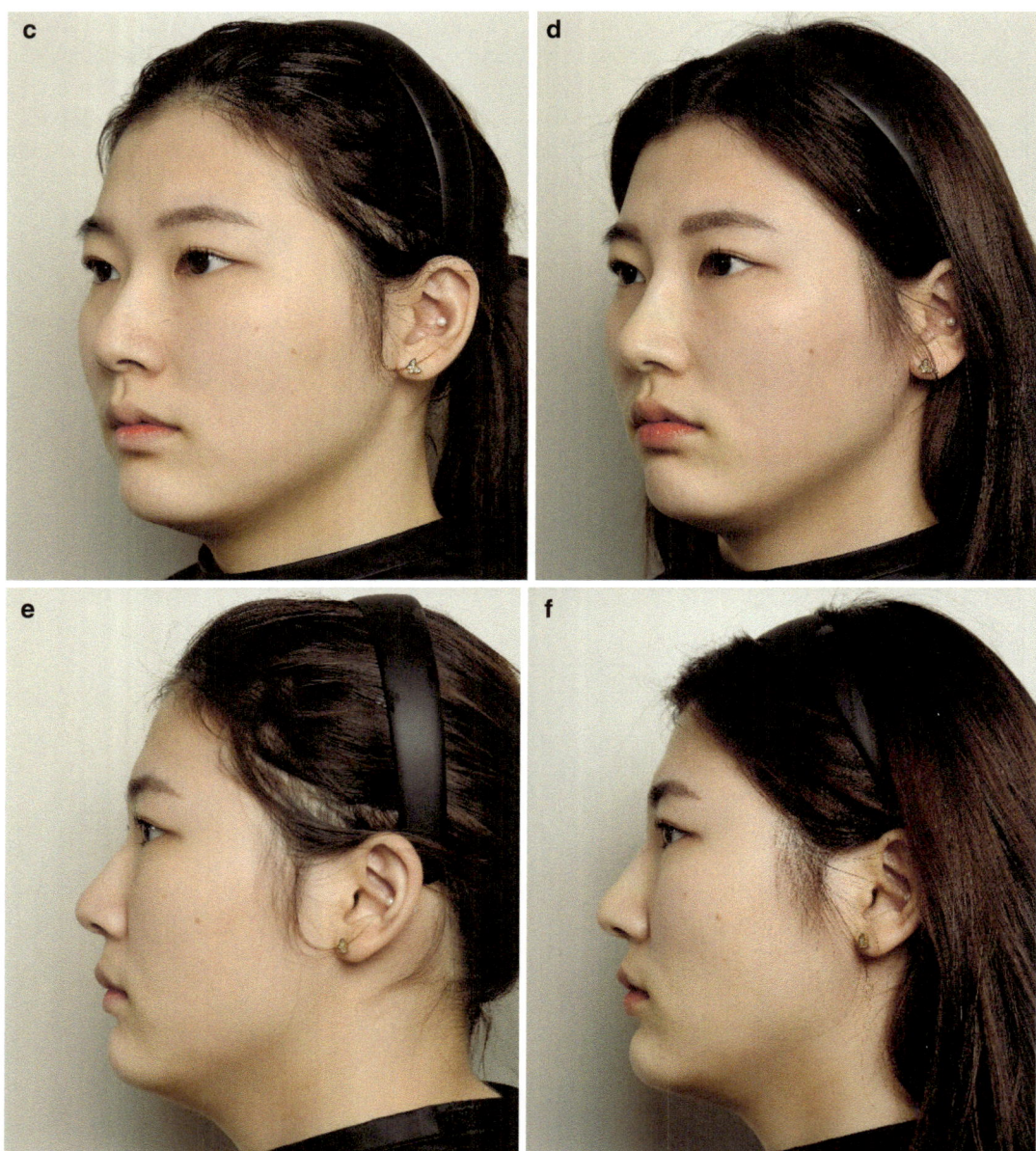

Fig. 6.12 (continued)

References

1. Scheuer JF 3rd, Sieber DA, Pezeshk RA, Gassman AA, Campbell CF, Rohrich RJ. Facial danger zones: techniques to maximize safety during soft-tissue filler injections. Plast Reconstr Surg. 2017 May;139(5):1103–8. https://doi.org/10.1097/PRS.0000000000003309.
2. Lee W, Kim JS, Oh W, Koh IS, Yang EJ. Nasal dorsum augmentation using soft tissue filler injection. J Cosmet Dermatol. 2019 Jun 3; https://doi.org/10.1111/jocd.13018.
3. Moon HJ. Injection rhinoplasty using filler. Facial Plast Surg Clin North Am. 2018 Aug;26(3):323–30. https://doi.org/10.1016/j.fsc.2018.03.006.
4. Choi DY, Bae JH, Youn KH, Kim W, Suwanchinda A, Tanvaa T, Kim HJ. Topography of the dorsal nasal artery and its clinical implications for augmentation of the dorsum of the nose. J Cosmet Dermatol. 2018 Aug;17(4):637–42. https://doi.org/10.1111/jocd.12720.
5. Beleznay K, Carruthers JD, Humphrey S, Jones D. Avoiding and treating blindness from fillers: a review of the world literature. Dermatol Surg. 2015 Oct;41(10):1097–117. https://doi.org/10.1097/DSS.0000000000000486.
6. Beleznay K, Carruthers JDA, Humphrey S, Carruthers A, Jones D. Update on avoiding and treating blindness from fillers: a recent review of the world literature. Aesthet Surg J. 2019 May 16;39(6):662–74. https://doi.org/10.1093/asj/sjz053.
7. Harb A, Brewster CT. The nonsurgical rhinoplasty: a retrospective review of 5000 treatments. Plast Reconstr Surg. 2020 Mar;145(3):661–7. https://doi.org/10.1097/PRS.0000000000006554.
8. Moon HJ, Lee W, Do Kim H, Lee IH, Kim SW. Doppler ultrasonographic anatomy of the midline nasal dorsum. Aesthet Plast Surg. 2021 Jun;45(3):1178–83. https://doi.org/10.1007/s00266-020-02025-1.
9. Lee Y, Oh SM, Lee W, Yang EJ. Comparison of hyaluronic acid filler ejection pressure with injection force for safe filler injection. J Cosmet Dermatol. 2021 May;20(5):1551–6. https://doi.org/10.1111/jocd.14064.
10. Lee W, Oh W, Moon HJ, Koh IS, Yang EJ. Soft tissue filler properties can be altered by a small-diameter needle. Dermatol Surg. 2020 Sep;46(9):1155–62. https://doi.org/10.1097/DSS.0000000000002220.
11. Kang SH, Moon SH, Kim HS. Nonsurgical rhinoplasty with polydioxanone threads and fillers. Dermatol Surg. 2020 May;46(5):664–70. https://doi.org/10.1097/DSS.0000000000002146.

The filler injection at the midface is usually performed in multiple locations at once. For example, the tear trough, anterior malar, and lateral cheek are corrected concomitantly. Consideration should be paid to the total amount of filler. Doctors should estimate the total amount of HA filler injection (Fig. 7.1). There are chances of delayed hypersensitivity when injecting a large amount.

7.1 Tear Trough Deformity

7.1.1 Anatomy

The nasojugal groove appears a complex structure with the tear trough ligament, orbital septal fat, and border between the preseptal portion and orbital portion of orbicularis oculi muscle [1]. The orbicularis retaining ligament can be divided into the medial side and lateral side by the mid-pupillary line and the medial side is a tighter and hard structure. This structure is called the tear trough ligament but its anatomical nomenclature is not defined. The medial side is composed of a tight structure because the orbicularis retaining ligament and zygomatico cutaneous ligament tend to aggregate at the medial side [2].

Also, grooves can be prominent because there is not much fat in the pretarsal or preseptal area, but subcutaneous fat exists in the orbital fat area. Sometimes the festoon is the cause of aging phe-

nomena [3]. When orbital fat is extruded, surgical removal by transconjunctival or transcutaneous procedure is needed. But if there is only a nasojugal groove, a filler injection can provide good results.

But when muscle fiber extends to the orbital rim tightly or the tear trough ligament is tightly attached, good aesthetic results cannot be performed. Then, a surgical correction would be the only solution [4]. Usually muscle fiber does not attach to the orbital rim, and a correction can be performed by HA filler injection.

Thus, the tear trough is not just a ligament but a complex deformity so an injection considering these factors is important. It is quite safe when an injection is performed at SOOF deeply, but the tear trough area would not have SOOF (Fig. 7.2), so considering the anatomical layer, a deep injection (between OOM and bone) and superficial injection (between OOM and skin) can be performed concomitantly. When injecting superficially, the Tyndall effect or nodule formation might occur, so a small amount of HA filler should be injected.

When performing a deep injection, the most important vessel would be the angular vein. It runs between the septal portion of the orbicularis oculi muscle and the LLS muscle, so it runs on the medial part of the tear trough. Doctors should consider the pathway of the angular vein.

The angular artery runs on the medial side of the angular vein at the tear trough area so it

Fig. 7.1 Midface
augmentation after
2 weeks. In total 3.9 mL
of hyaluronic acid filler
was injected

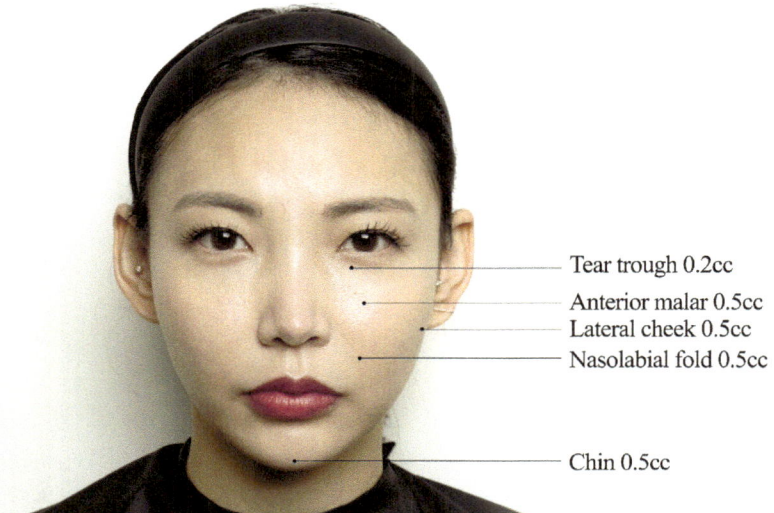

Tear trough 0.2cc

Anterior malar 0.5cc
Lateral cheek 0.5cc
Nasolabial fold 0.5cc

Chin 0.5cc

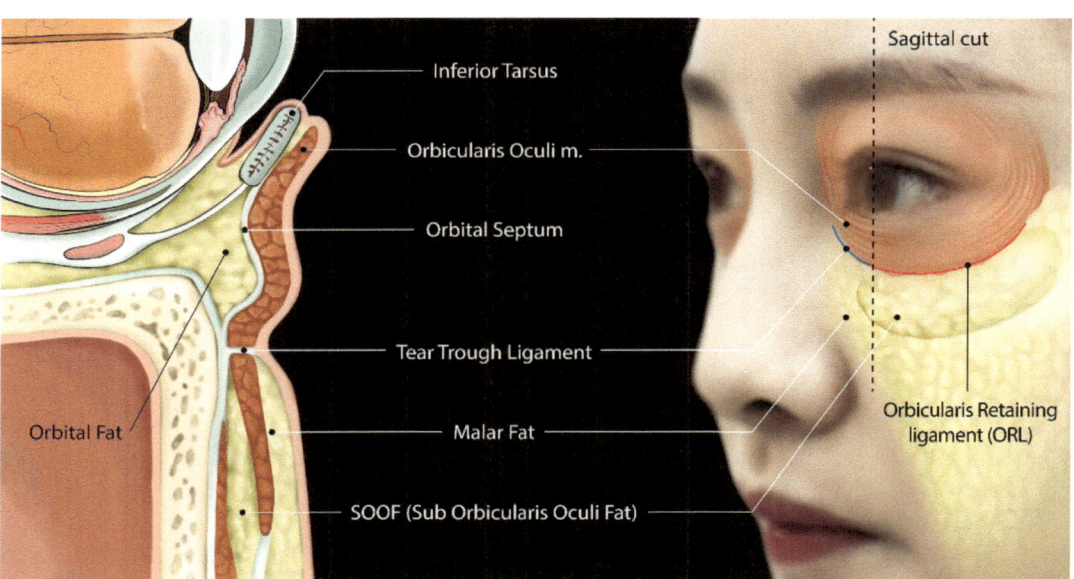

Fig. 7.2 Tear trough ligament and surrounding structures

is relatively safe where the angular artery branches from the detoured branch of the facial artery. The facial artery runs toward the inferior orbital artery and anastomosis with the angular artery, so the angular artery might be located in a very similar position to the angular vein, so extreme caution is needed (Figs. 7.3 and 7.4) [5].

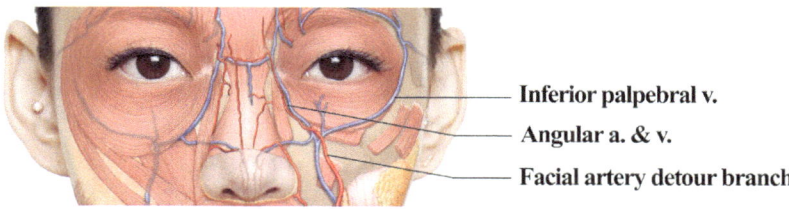

Inferior palpebral v.

Angular a. & v.

Facial artery detour branch

Fig. 7.3 Angular artery and vein pathway. The angular artery runs on the medial side of the angular vein (Rt), the angular artery (from detoured branch of facial artery) runs similar to the angular vein (Lt)

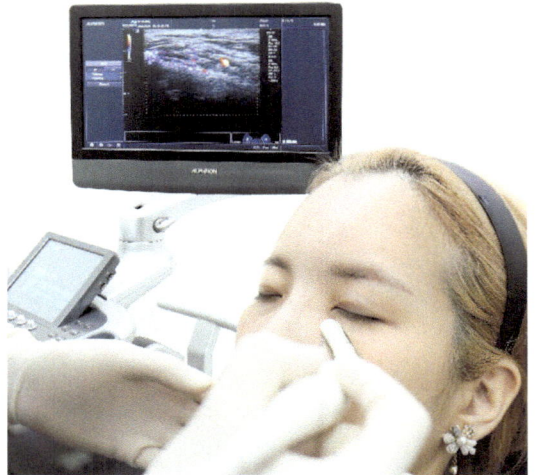

Fig. 7.4 Doppler ultrasound finding of angular artery at tear trough area

7.1.2   Filler Choice

Lifting capacity is relatively unimportant. High cohesiveness is needed (Table 7.1). The injected filler at the tear trough lasts longer compared to other sites. The causes might be relatively less movement of muscle in this area or that there is relatively less hyaluronidase in this area but it is not defined. In our experience, the duration is more than a year [6].

7.1.3   Anesthesia

Topical anesthesia is usually performed due to precise injection (Fig. 7.5). An infraorbital regional nerve block is not usually performed because it might result in temporary swelling and might affect the filler injection procedure.

7.1.4   Needle Versus Cannula

As previously described in anatomy, there is a risk of interrupting the angular artery or angular vein so it is safer to use a cannula. Always consider the Tyndall effect when injecting superficially [7].

7.1.5   Injection Technique (Figs. 7.6, 7.7, 7.8, 7.9, and 7.10)

Table 7.1 Rheological test result of Lorient filler

Product	G′ (Pa)	G″ (Pa)	Complex viscosity (μ)	Tan delta	Cohesiveness (N)
Lorient No. 2	203	41	1,673,007	0.20	0.4401
Lorient No. 4	338	95	2,795,776	0.28	0.4237
Lorient No. 6	413	121	3,423,232	0.29	0.4454

The author uses No. 2 for tear trough correction

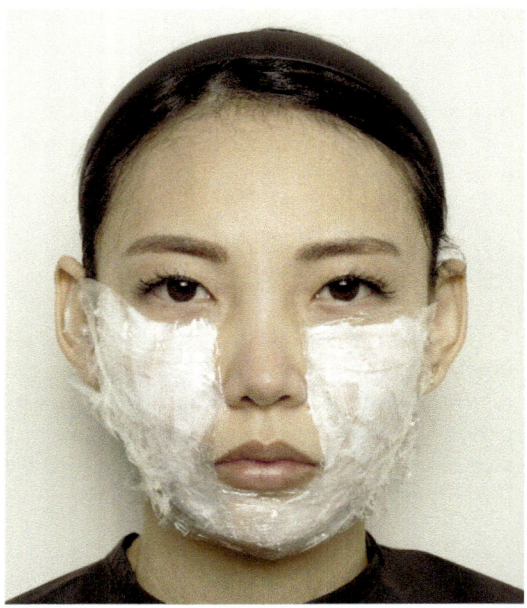

Fig. 7.5 Topical anesthesia cream

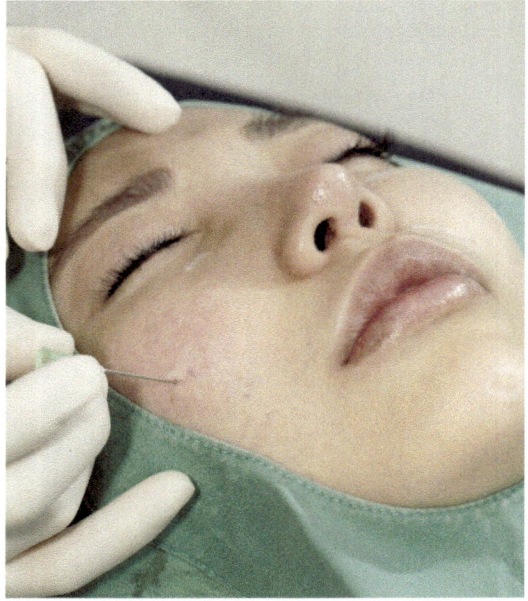

Fig. 7.7 21G needle puncture

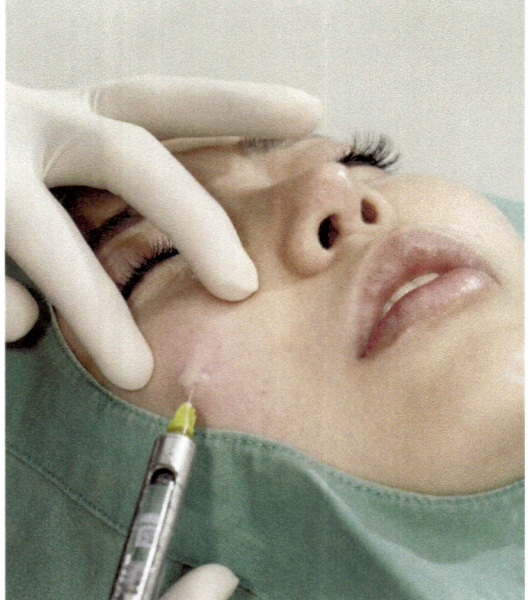

Fig. 7.6 Local anesthesia at the entry point

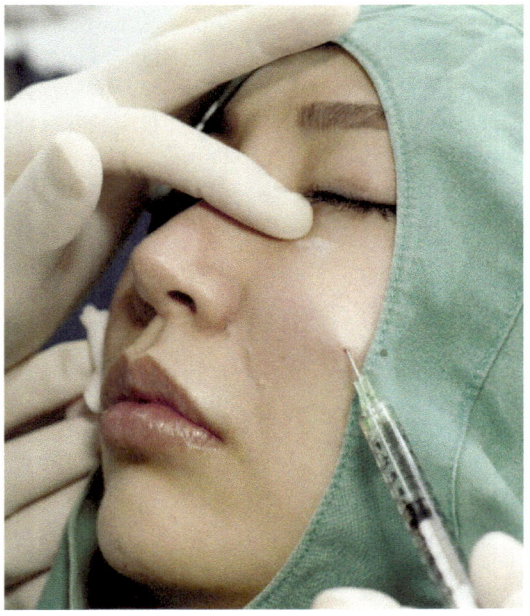

Fig. 7.8 Change to upright position, locate cannula tip to desired layer and inject precisely

7.2 Anterior Malar Augmentation

7.2.1 Anatomy and General Considerations

One of the largest differences in terms of aesthetic opinion between Western and Oriental anatomy might be the malar area and mandibular angle area. Oriental females like to have a smooth contour at the zygomatic arch area because of

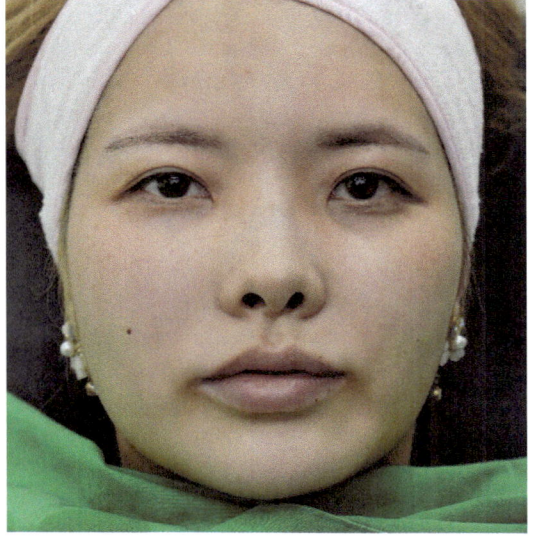

Fig. 7.9 Comparison between right side (finished procedure) and left side (not injected)

feminization. A relatively prominent anterior malar area for prominent contour. So, there is a difference of opinion and some Western concepts such as hinderer's line cannot explain the Oriental patient's needs [8].

In the aspect of Western patients, a prominent cheekbone is considered youthful in appearance but for Oriental patients, the anterior malar area should be more prominent. Thus, augmentation of the malar portion near the inferior orbital rim is needed.

This area is below the orbicularis retaining ligament, so when performing an anterior malar augmentation, doctors should consider the orbicularis retaining ligament and zygomatico cutaneous ligament.

7.2.2 Injection Technique

Multiple structures are located. When performing a deep injection behind the orbicularis oculi muscle, the target should be the prezygomatic space, the deep malar fat pad including SOOF. But there are some dangerous structures. Always keep in mind the infraorbital artery and nerve. The facial artery detoured branch should be considered. The angular vein and inferior palpebral vein anastomosis to the facial vein in this area, which should be considered (Fig. 7.11) [9]. So the author always uses a cannula.

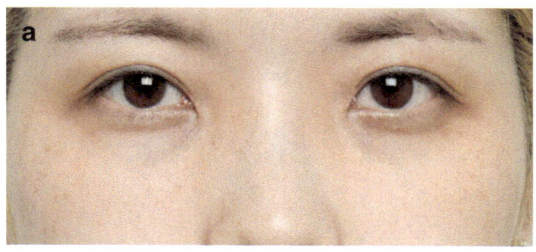
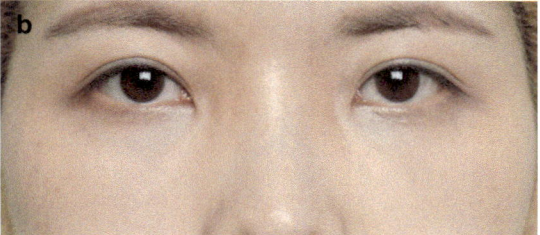

Fig. 7.10 Tear trough deformity correction Lorient No. 2 0.3 mL (**a**) Preinjection and (**b**) Postinjection

Fig. 7.11 Vessel anatomy of anterior malar area

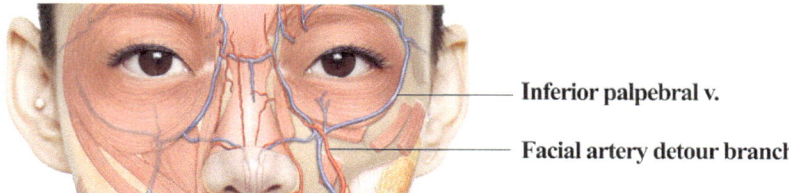

Inferior palpebral v.

Facial artery detour branch

Various vessels are located so gentle injection by cannula is most important. The target of this area is the deep malar fat pad and prezygomatic space so better not to inject by touching the bone [10]. The entry point is the same as for tear trough correction (Figs. 7.6 and 7.7) and inject in the upright position (Fig. 7.12).

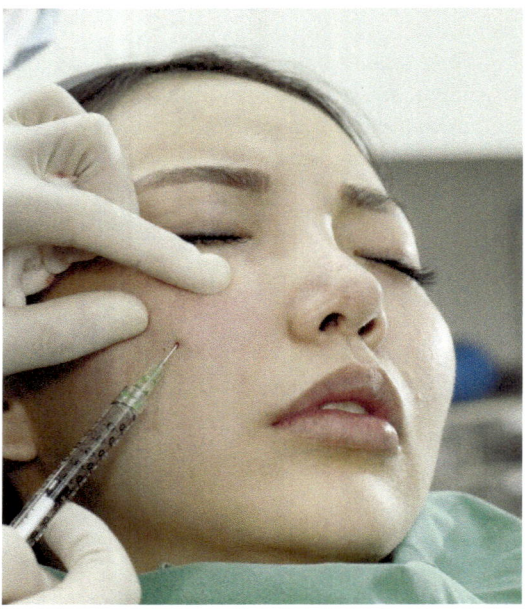

Fig. 7.12 Anterior malar augmentation injection

7.2.3   Filler Choice

A relatively high lifting capacity filler is needed because of augmentation under muscle (Table 7.2).

7.3   Lateral Cheek Correction

There are abundant fibrous bands between the skin and SMAS in the lateral cheek area. Because of fibrous bands, the filler might migrate to undesired spaces. Thus, injecting in an upright position is recommended. When performing using a cannula, making small spaces by feeling to cut fibrous bands will help the procedure (Fig. 7.13).

This area is enough to fill the superficial fat compartment which is lateral to temporal cheek fat. A deep injection is not needed for aesthetic contour and risk of parotid duct or facial nerve damage.

The transverse facial artery is from the superficial temporal artery or external carotid artery and runs between and under the zygomatic arch and parotid duct, so when correcting lateral cheeks, the artery can be encountered. But since the space is not limited, there is not much chance of vascular injury. Several variations should be considered including reaching the dorsal nasal artery, so a gentle injection is always needed [11].

Table 7.2 Rheologic Lorient test results

Product	G′ (Pa)	G″ (Pa)	Complex viscosity (μ)	Tan delta	Cohesiveness (N)
Lorient No. 2	203	41	1,673,007	0.20	0.4401
Lorient No. 4	338	95	2,795,776	0.28	0.4237
Lorient No. 6	413	121	3,423,232	0.29	0.4454

The author uses No. 4 or No. 6 for anterior malar augmentation

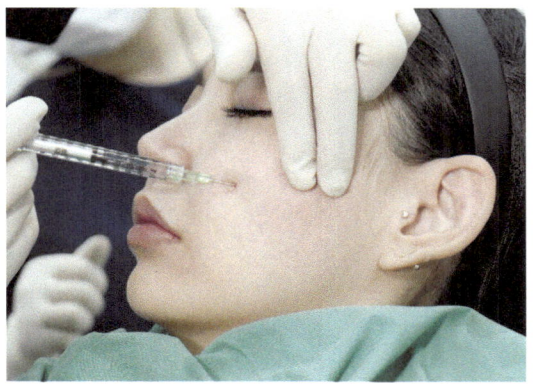

The author uses Lorient No. 2 or No. 4 for correcting lateral cheek depression.

Fig. 7.13 Correction of lateral cheek depression

7.4   Tear Trough, Anterior Malar Augmentation, Lateral Cheek Correction Pre and Postprocedural Photograph (Fig. 7.14)

a

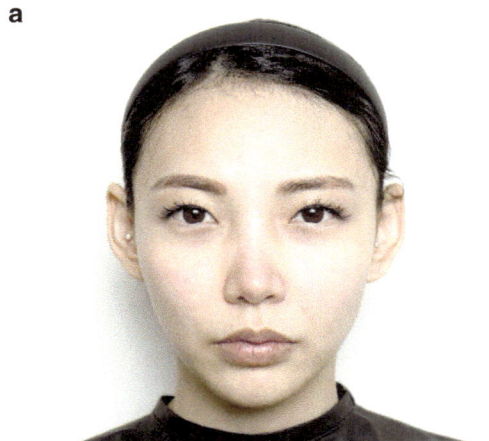
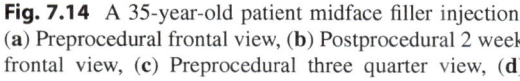

b

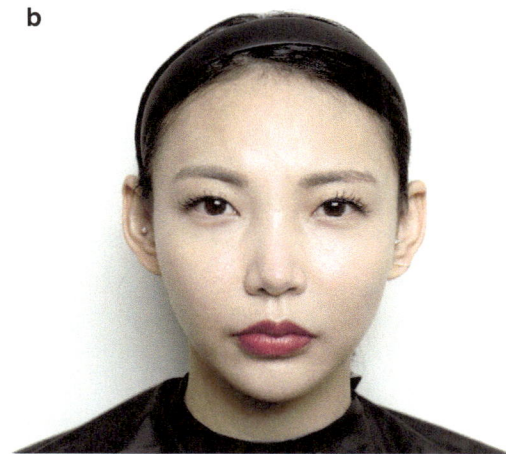

Fig. 7.14 A 35-year-old patient midface filler injection. (**a**) Preprocedural frontal view, (**b**) Postprocedural 2 week frontal view, (**c**) Preprocedural three quarter view, (**d**) Postprocedural 2 week three quarter view, (**e**) Preprocedural lateral view, and (**f**) Postprocedural 2 week lateral view

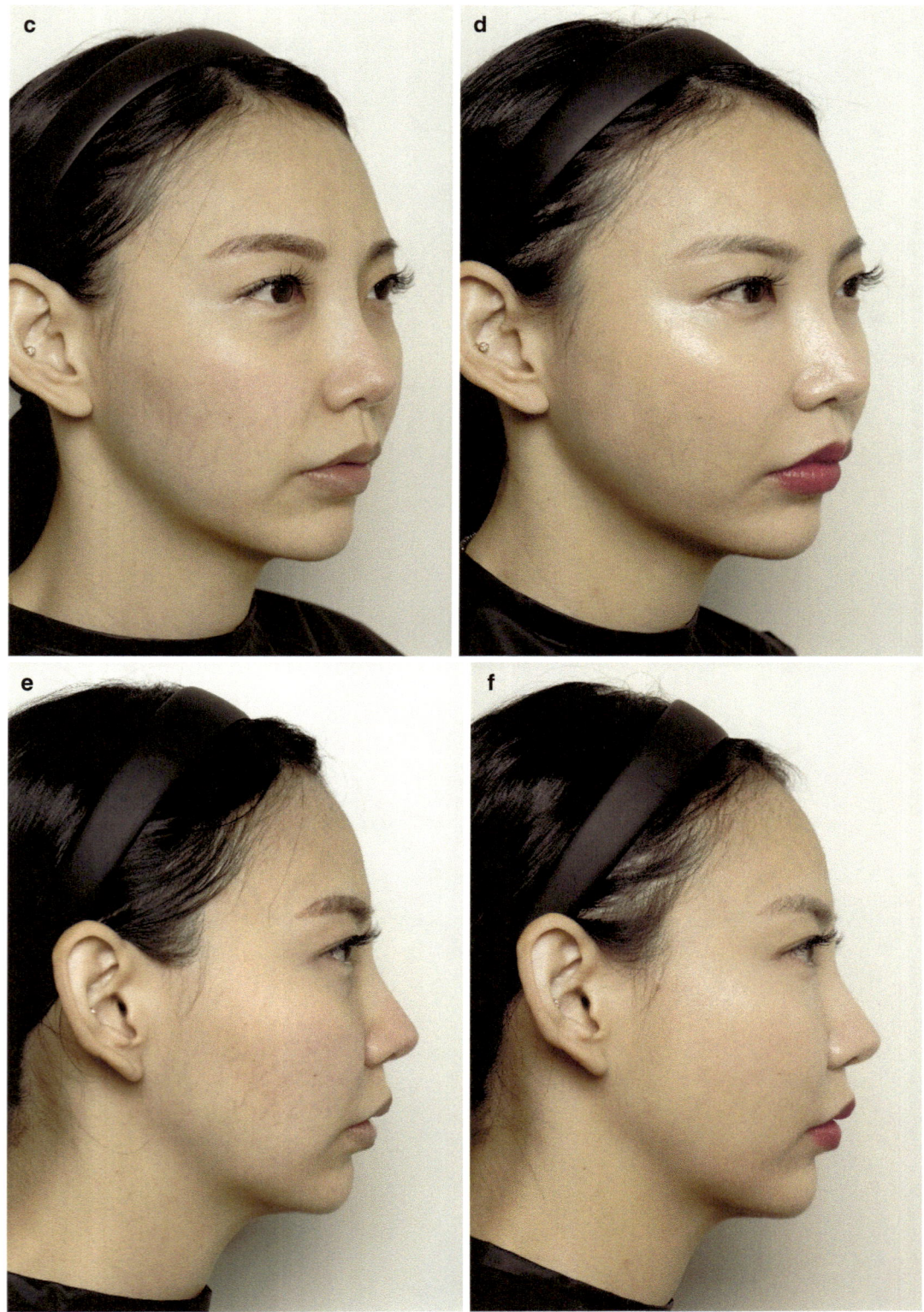

Fig. 7.14 (continued)

References

1. Lee JH, Hong G. Definitions of groove and hollowness of the infraorbital region and clinical treatment using soft-tissue filler. Arch Plast Surg. 2018;45:214–21.

2. Wong CH, Mendelson B. Facial soft-tissue spaces and retaining ligaments of the midcheek: defining the premaxillary space. Plast Reconstr Surg. 2013 Jul;132(1):49–56. https://doi.org/10.1097/PRS.0b013e3182910a57.

3. Kpodzo DS, Nahai F, McCord CD. Malar mounds and festoons: review of current management. Aesthet Surg J. 2014 Feb;34(2):235–48. https://doi.org/10.1177/1090820X13517897.

4. Lee W, Cho JK, Koh IS, Kim HM, Yang EJ. Infraorbital groove correction by microfat injection after lower blepharoplasty. J Plast Reconstr Aesthet Surg. 2020 Apr;73(4):777–82. https://doi.org/10.1016/j.bjps.2019.11.016.

5. Kim YS, Choi DY, Gil YC, Hu KS, Tansatit T, Kim HJ. The anatomical origin and course of the angular artery regarding its clinical implications. Dermatol Surg. 2014 Oct;40(10):1070–6. https://doi.org/10.1097/01.DSS.0000452661.61916.b5.

6. Landau M. Hyaluronidase caveats in treating filler complications. Dermatol Surg. 2015 Dec;41(Suppl 1):S347–53. https://doi.org/10.1097/DSS.0000000000000555.

7. DeLorenzi C. Complications of injectable fillers, part I. Aesthet Surg J. 2013 May;33(4):561–75. https://doi.org/10.1177/1090820X13484492.

8. Shamban A, Clague MD, von Grote E, Nogueira A. A novel and more aesthetic injection pattern for malar cheek volume restoration. Aesthet Plast Surg. 2018 Feb;42(1):197–200. https://doi.org/10.1007/s00266-017-0981-1.

9. Lee SH, Lee HJ, Kim YS, Tansatit T, Kim HJ. Novel anatomic description of the course of the inferior palpebral vein for minimally invasive aesthetic treatments. Dermatol Surg. 2016 May;42(5):618–23. https://doi.org/10.1097/DSS.0000000000000700.

10. Mendelson BC, Jacobson SR. Surgical anatomy of the midcheek: facial layers, spaces, and the midcheek segments. Clin Plast Surg. 2008 Jul;35(3):395–404; discussion 393. https://doi.org/10.1016/j.cps.2008.02.003.

11. Toure G, Nguyen TM, Vlavonou S, Ndiaye MM. Transverse facial artery: its role in blindness after cosmetic filler and botulinum toxin injections. J Plast Reconstr Aesthet Surg. 2020 Dec 24:S1748-6815(20)30717-8. https://doi.org/10.1016/j.bjps.2020.12.042.

8.1 General Considerations

The nasolabial fold correction is one of the most common filler injection procedures. When new fillers arrive on the market, WSRS (Wrinkle severity rate scale) correction scores in articles are utilized to prove the effectiveness of the filler. There are some scores for wrinkle corrections which are WSRS, GAIS (Global Aesthetic Improvement Scale), VAS (Visual Analogue Scale), and FACE Q. But these parameters are variable by doctor and/or patient and the most commonly used WSRS was made in 2004 (Fig. 8.1) [1] so more objective parameters might be needed.

The WSRS grade 5 case also combines cheek skin drooping so other procedures such as lifting are needed for better aesthetic results.

One of the causes of various types of nasolabial fold is the descent of nasolabial fat (superficial fat compartment) [2]. The aging process results in sagging of superficial fat and a decrease in dermal elasticity [3]. This is the reason why the nasolabial fold disappears when the patient lays down.

Another cause is the diminishing volume of deep medial cheek fat. The aging process decreases the volume of the deep fat component and causes a deep nasolabial fold [4]. This is one of the main reasons to inject at the deep medial cheek fat. Between the deep medial cheek fat and periosteum is called Ristow's Space [4] and the

theory of the 1 cm space is the same as the deep pyriform space [5] but the author thinks Ristow's Space is a kind of surgical potential space. And it is the first target to correct the nasolabial fold.

Another cause of nasolabial folds is the repetitive movement of muscles attached to the dermal layer of the nasolabial fold. These are the so-called lip elevators which are the levator labii superioris alaque nasi (LLSAN), levator labii superioris, zygomaticus major, and zygomaticus minor [6]. So, consideration should be made of a botulinum toxin injection if the nasolabial fold is severe.

Since there are multiple proposed causes of nasolabial folds, a successful correction is needed by understanding deep layer correction, superficial layer correction, correlation with vessels, and the relationship with mimetic muscles.

8.2 Anatomy

The arterial pathway of the facial artery is most important (Fig. 8.2). The facial artery runs the same as the nasolabial fold (Fig. 8.3) but there are some variations such as the detoured branch which runs toward the infraorbital foramen and also a variation of layers that are located under muscle or over muscle [7]. Generally, the supraperiosteal layer is known for being a safe injection layer but there are variations so it is not 100% safe [8]. Always remember the variations

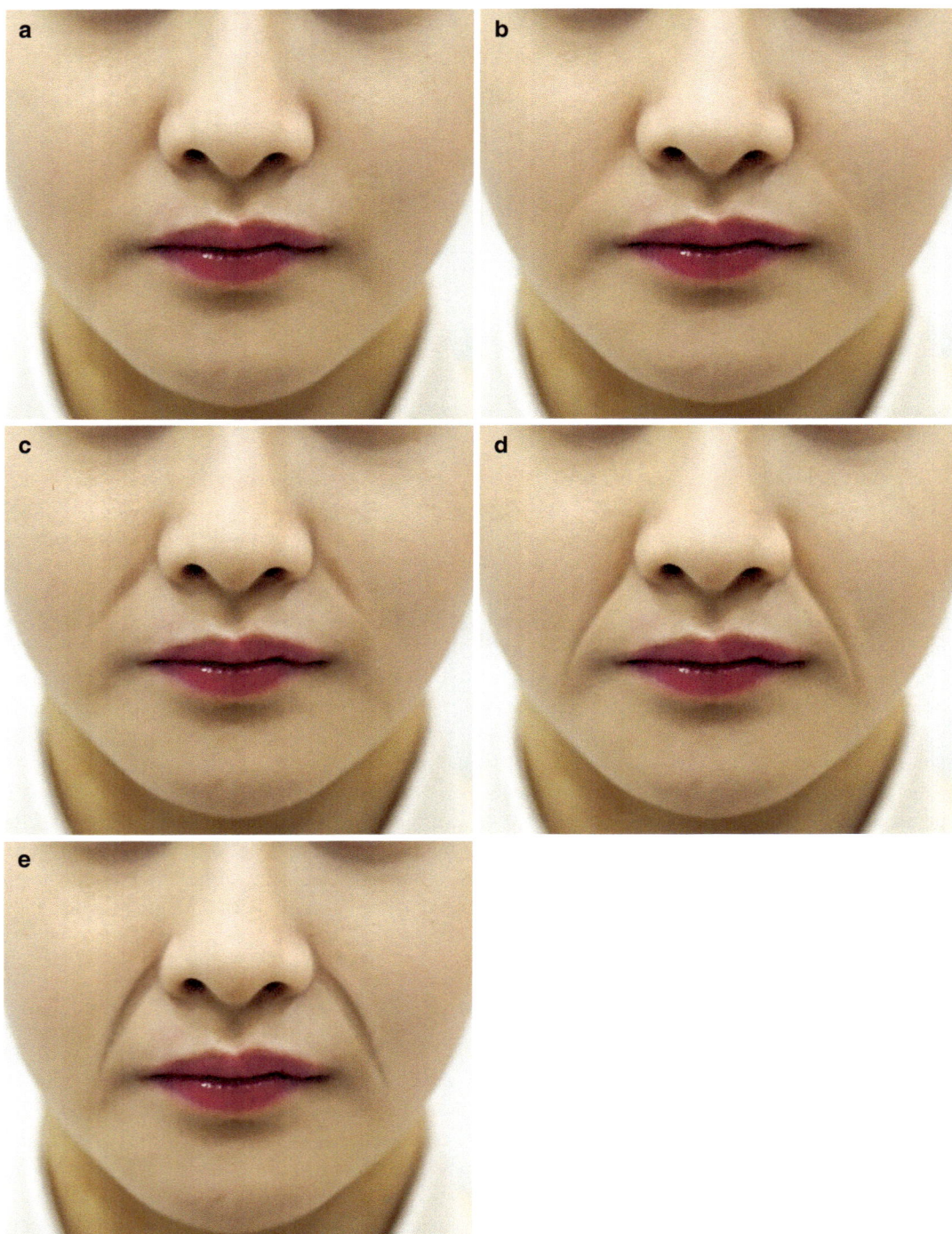

Fig. 8.1 (**a**) WSRS grade 1: (absent). (**b**) WSRS grade 2: (mild) shallow but visible. (**c**) WSRS grade 3: (moderate). (**d**) WSRS grade 4: (severe) long and deep. (**e**) WSRS grade 5: (extreme)

Fig. 8.2 Vascular anatomy at nasolabial fold. Facial artery can be located at nasolabial fold (Rt) and facial artery can detour from nasolabial fold (Lt)

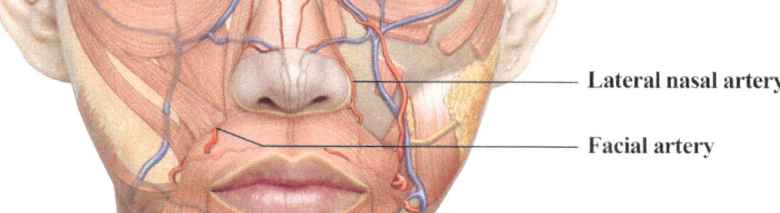

— Lateral nasal artery

— Facial artery

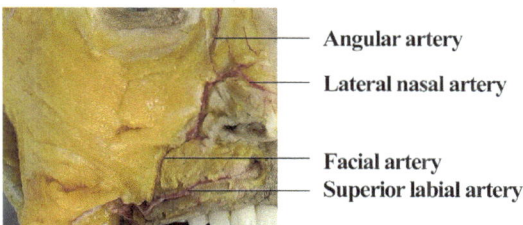

— Angular artery
— Lateral nasal artery

— Facial artery
— Superior labial artery

Fig. 8.3 Cadaveric anatomy at nasolabial fold area

and inject little by little very gently. A recent study has shown that using a Doppler ultrasound is a good tool to prevent vascular complications.

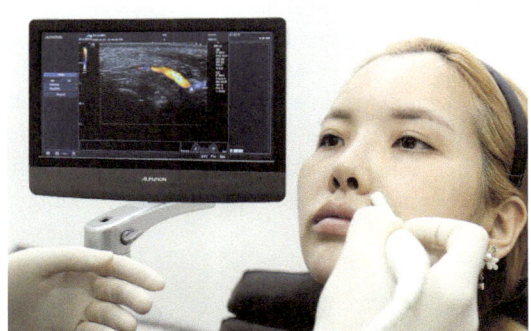

Fig. 8.4 Doppler ultrasound probe detection

8.3   Doppler Ultrasound

All the layers including the bony layer at the nasolabial fold can be detected by ultrasound frequency 8 ~ 10 MHz, and the facial artery is a relatively large diameter vessel so it is detected easily (Figs. 8.4 and 8.5).

8.4   Filler Choice

Lifting the nasolabial fold is the main purpose of a filler injection but mimetic muscles are continuously moving so tissue integration is important. Gel hardness should be considered when injecting deep or shallow (Table 8.1).

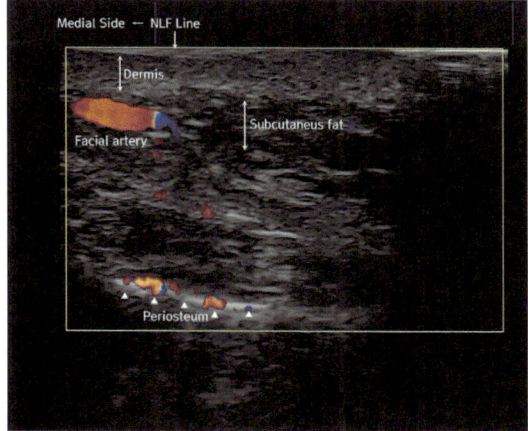

Fig. 8.5 Facial artery is detected at subcutaneous layer

8.5   Cannula Versus Needle

When performing by cannula, the entry point which is made for augmenting the anterior malar area can be used. A superaperiosteal layer injec-

tion is possible. But even if the deep layer is corrected, skin indentation can appear and a subdermal injection might be performed by needle. A subdermal injection can be performed with a cannula using a skin tenting technique. A dual plane injection provides better results but doctors should never inject into the subcutaneous layer.

Table 8.1   Rheologic test results of Lorient HA filler

Product	G′ (Pa)	G″ (Pa)	Complex viscosity (μ)	Tan delta	Cohesiveness (N)
Lorient No. 2	203	41	1,673,007	0.20	0.4401
Lorient No. 4	338	95	2,795,776	0.28	0.4237
Lorient No. 6	413	121	3,423,232	0.29	0.4454

The author usually uses No. 4 and in cases of deep fold, uses No. 6. For subdermal injection, No. 2 is used

There should not be too much confidence in using a cannula. A thin cannula is like a needle [9]. And when using a cannula, doctors should also always consider the layer which is the deep layer. It is important not to inject at the nasolabial fat compartment. The needle perpendicular injection technique is another good technique unless the facial artery is not detected by Doppler ultrasound.

8.6   General Considerations

A lot of doctors forget to ask patients about previous surgery or previous filler injections. Silicone implants can be inserted into nasolabial folds and permanent fillers might have been injected previously. When a patient has previous operation history, only a small amount of subdermal injection can be performed.

One of the most important elements of nasolabial fold correction is not to correct too much a high level of nasolabial fold. The lateral nasal artery from the facial artery tends to be located at the subcutaneous layer and when performing with a high level of folds to correct alar recess, there might be risk of vascular complications.

8.7   Techniques (Figs. 8.6, 8.7, and 8.8)

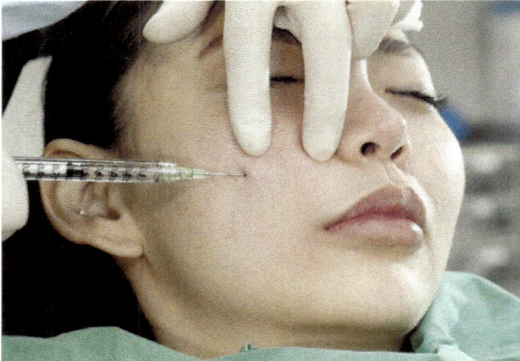

Fig. 8.6   Using the same entry point as for anterior malar augmentation, the cannula tip is located at the supraperiosteal layer by touching the bony area and then injecting gently

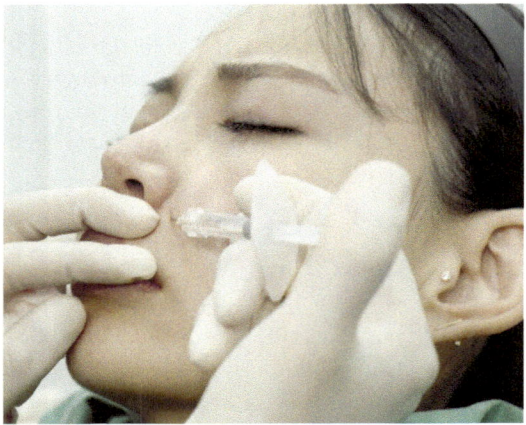

Fig. 8.7   A small amount of subdermal injection. Lorient No. 2 is used for shallow wrinkles

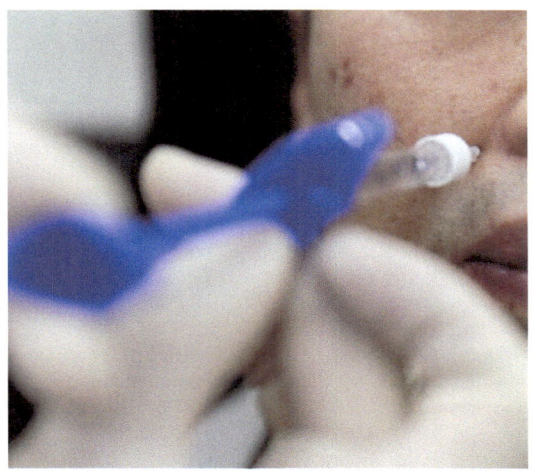

Fig. 8.8 Deep bolus injection. A Doppler ultrasound test should be performed before injection and the aspiration test should be performed [10]

8.8   Pre- and Postprocedural Photograph (Figs. 8.9 and 8.10)

8.9   Vascular Complications

An intravascular embolism in the facial artery can cause skin necrosis and/or ocular complications (Fig. 8.11).

The most important factor for prognosis of skin necrosis is treatment time. When treatment time is delayed, a nasal scar might develop and sometimes alar retraction develops [11]. Injecting hyaluronidase as soon as possible is the best treatment for revascularization [12]. A report

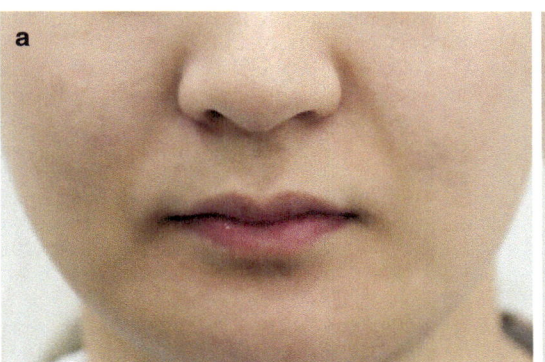
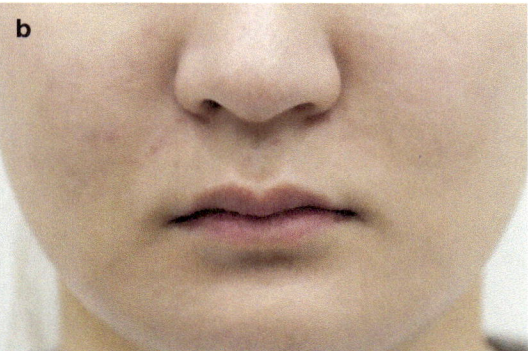

Fig. 8.9 A 27-year-old female patient 1 mL injected each. (**a**) Preprocedural and (**b**) Postprocedural 2 weeks

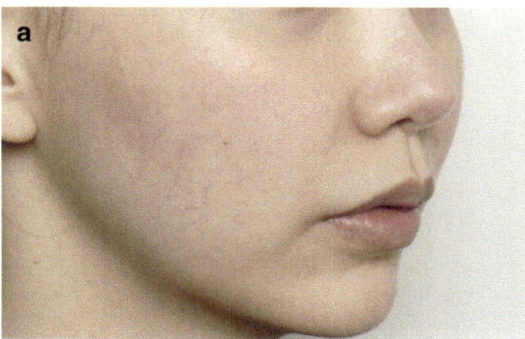
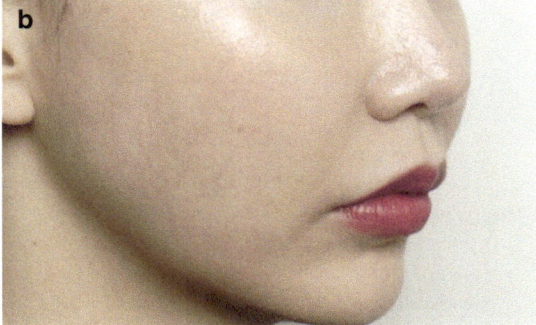

Fig. 8.10 A 35-year-old female patient 0.5 mL injected each. (**a**) Preprocedural and (**b**) Postprocedural 2 weeks

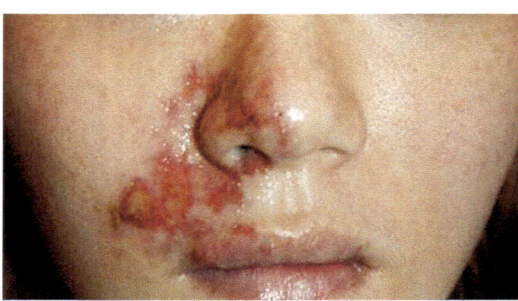

Fig. 8.11 Two days after HA filler injection-induced skin necrosis

shows the treatment should start in the first three days [13].

Important factors to consider injecting hyaluronidase for skin necrosis.

1. Inject hyaluronidase as soon as possible. An emergency call should be made even on the weekend.
2. A high enough dose is needed. Guess which vessel is involved and more than 100 IU at 1 point should be injected at a 1-cm distance. For example, if skin necrosis is discovered after a nasolabial fold correction, hyaluronidase should be injected into all involved areas such as the forehead supratrochlear territory, nasal alar lateral nasal artery territory, and nasolabial facial artery territory.
3. Inject repetitively for 30 mins to 1 hour. Hyaluronic acid filler does not degrade immediately by hyaluronidase.
4. Subcutaneous injection not intravenous or intraarterial.

References

1. Day DJ, Littler CM, Swift RW, Gottlieb S. The wrinkle severity rating scale: a validation study. Am J Clin Dermatol. 2004;5(1):49–52.
2. Gierloff M, Stöhring C, Buder T, Gassling V, Açil Y, Wiltfang J. Aging changes of the midfacial fat compartments: a computed tomographic study. Plast Reconstr Surg. 2012 Jan;129(1):263–73. https://doi.org/10.1097/PRS.0b013e3182362b96.
3. Ezure T, Amano S. Involvement of upper cheek sagging in nasolabial fold formation. Skin Res Technol. 2012 Aug;18(3):259–64. https://doi.org/10.1111/j.1600-0846.2011.00567.x.
4. Rohrich RJ, Pessa JE, Ristow B. The youthful cheek and the deep medial fat compartment. Plast Reconstr Surg. 2008 Jun;121(6):2107–12. https://doi.org/10.1097/PRS.0b013e31817123c6.
5. Surek CK, Vargo J, Lamb J. Deep pyriform space: anatomical clarifications and clinical implications. Plast Reconstr Surg. 2016 Jul;138(1):59–64. https://doi.org/10.1097/PRS.0000000000002262.
6. Beer GM, Manestar M, Mihic-Probst D. The causes of the nasolabial crease: a histomorphological study. Clin Anat. 2013 Mar;26(2):196–203. https://doi.org/10.1002/ca.22100.
7. Lee JG, Yang HM, Choi YJ, Favero V, Kim YS, Hu KS, et al. Facial arterial depth and relationship with the facial musculature layer. Plast Reconstr Surg. 2015;135(2):437–44.
8. Lee W, Kim JS, Moon HJ, Yang EJ. A safe Doppler ultrasound-guided method for nasolabial fold correction with hyaluronic acid filler. Aesthet Surg J. 2021 May 18;41(6):NP486–92. https://doi.org/10.1093/asj/sjaa153.
9. Pavicic T, Webb KL, Frank K, Gotkin RH, Tamura B, Cotofana S. Arterial wall penetration forces in needles versus cannulas. Plast Reconstr Surg. 2019 Mar;143(3):504e–512e. https://doi.org/10.1097/PRS.0000000000005321.
10. Moon HJ, Lee W, Kim JS, Yang EJ, Sundaram H. Aspiration revisited: prospective evaluation of a physiologically pressurized model with animal correlation and broader applicability to filler complications. Aesthet Surg J. 2021 Apr 16:sjab194. https://doi.org/10.1093/asj/sjab194.
11. Grunebaum LD, Bogdan Allemann I, Dayan S, Mandy S, Baumann L. The risk of alar necrosis associated with dermal filler injection. Dermatol Surg. 2009 Oct;35(Suppl 2):1635–40. https://doi.org/10.1111/j.1524-4725.2009.01342.x.
12. DeLorenzi C. New high dose pulsed hyaluronidase protocol for hyaluronic acid filler vascular adverse events. Aesthet Surg J. 2017 Jul 1;37(7):814–25. https://doi.org/10.1093/asj/sjw251.
13. Hong JY, Seok J, Ahn GR, Jang YJ, Li K, Kim BJ. Impending skin necrosis after dermal filler injection: a "golden time" for first-aid intervention. Dermatol Ther. 2017 Mar;30(2). https://doi.org/10.1111/dth.12440

9.1 Marionette Lines

Marionette lines (labiomandibular fold) are different from the nasolabial fold. Usually what appears is skin drooping at the premasseteric space. Compared to the nasolabial fold, it is difficult to correct WRSR 4,5 only by filler because of skin drooping but marionette lines usually combine skin drooping and/or superior jowl fat compartment drooping so the limitation of procedure should be explained to the patient before injection [1].

The mandibular retaining ligament is known as a true ligament which is attached from the mandible to skin and plays an important role in formation of the fold. So a filler injection combining the correction of skin drooping makes for a better aesthetic result (Fig. 9.1) [2]. The relationship with the perioral muscles, which are the orbicularis oris, zygomaticus major, risorius, platysma, and depressor anguli oris should also be considered.

A high elasticity filler is not needed, but it is better to have a highly cohesive filler (Table 9.1).

The facial artery usually runs laterally from the marionette line. The inferior labial artery is usually located deep in muscle (Figs. 9.2 and 9.3). A marionette line injection is usually performed at the subcutaneous layer [3].

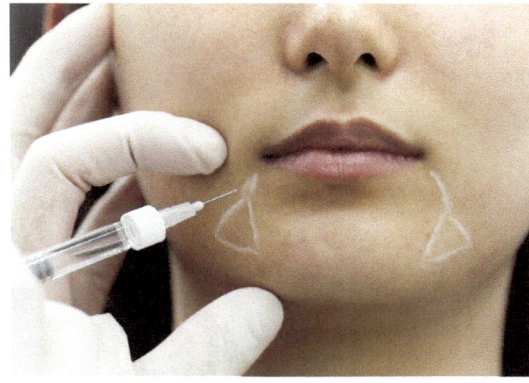

Fig. 9.1 Marionette line injection

9.2 Chin Augmentation

Rickettes line is the virtual line from the nose tip to chin [4]. With the mouth protruding or retracting, Rickettes line is important for the aesthetic aspect. The operation is usually performed via genioplasty or prosthesis insertion. Compared to an operation, a filler injection is an extremely easy procedure and a small amount of filler can make a more attractive face. It is important to decide whether the filler injection will perform projection or elongation of the chin. But too much chin elongation might result in the witch's chin phenomena, which should be considered.

© The Author(s), under exclusive license to Springer Nature Singapore Pte Ltd. 2022
W. Lee, *Safe Filler Injection Techniques*, https://doi.org/10.1007/978-981-16-6855-5_9

Table 9.1 Rheological test results of Lorient HA filler

Product	G′ (Pa)	G″ (Pa)	Complex viscosity (μ)	Tan delta	Cohesiveness (N)
Lorient No. 2	203	41	1,673,007	0.20	0.4401
Lorient No. 4	338	95	2,795,776	0.28	0.4237
Lorient No. 6	413	121	3,423,232	0.29	0.4454

The author uses No. 2 or No. 4 for marionette lines

Fig. 9.2 Relationship between inferior labial artery and marionette line

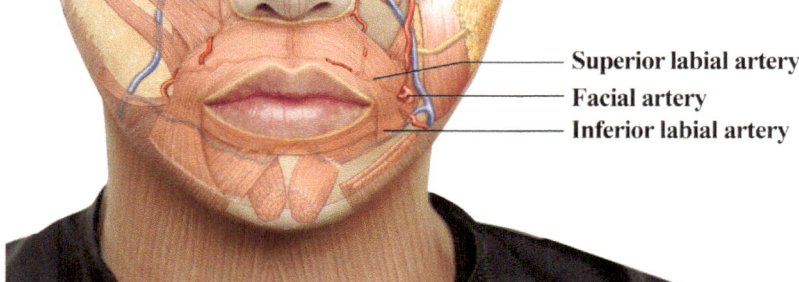

Superior labial artery
Facial artery
Inferior labial artery

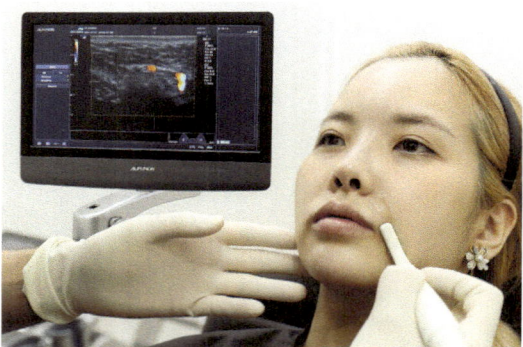

Fig. 9.3 Doppler ultrasound finding of marionette line

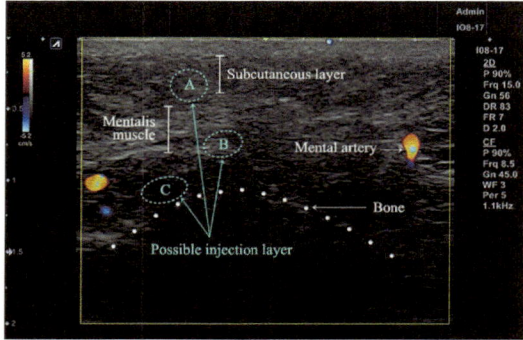

Fig. 9.4 Ultrasound finding of chin area and possible layer of chin augmentation. (A) Superficial fat (mental fat compartment), (B) Submentalis layer (submentalis fat), and (C) Supraperiosteal layer (submentalis fat)

The chin is a relatively safe location to inject but doctors should consider the relationship with the mentalis and perioral muscles. The mentalis muscle supports the lower lip and hyperactivity of the mentalis muscle can make a cobblestone appearance. So, it is suggested to inject botulinum toxin together.

The mentalis muscle starts from the incisive fossa of the mandible and is attached to the skin with a midline crossing as a cone shape appearance [5]. The lower part of the mentalis muscle decussates at the midline and submentalis fat exists between muscle and mandible [6]. This will be the target of the HA filler injection but considering the action of the mentalis, a high elastic filler is preferred. Also, a large amount of filler is not recommended because of granuloma formation [7]. The relationship between granuloma and bone resorption is not scientifically proven but injecting multiple layers is recommended (Fig. 9.4) [8].

Filler choice: A high G′ filler is needed such as nose injection (Table 9.2).

Technique: A perpendicular midline injection by needle is a very useful technique and is easy to make a chin shape. The submental artery branch might ascend at the midline and a cannula can be used after making the entry point lateral from the midline. The most important factor is whether projection or elongation is needed and making

Table 9.2 Rheological test of Lorient HA filler

Product	G′ (Pa)	G″ (Pa)	Complex viscosity (μ)	Tan delta	Cohesiveness (N)
Lorient No. 2	203	41	1,673,007	0.20	0.4401
Lorient No. 4	338	95	2,795,776	0.28	0.4237
Lorient No. 6	413	121	3,423,232	0.29	0.4454

The author uses No. 6 for chin augmentation

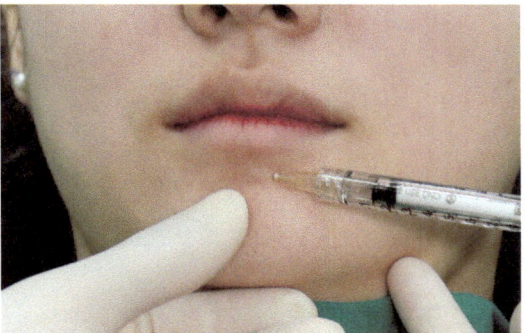

Fig. 9.5 Labiomental crease correction

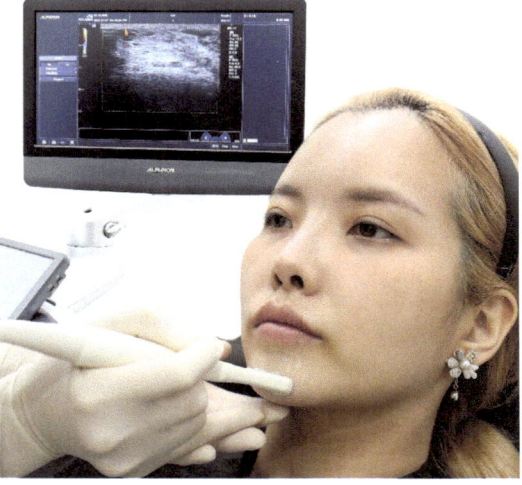

Fig. 9.6 Doppler ultrasound finding of chin

appropriate symmetry. When a labiomental groove appears between chin and lower lip, a low elastic filler can be injected at the subcutaneous layer (Fig. 9.5) [9].

The submental artery from the facial artery, inferior labial artery from facial artery and mental artery from external carotid artery make anastomosis at the chin area (Fig. 9.6) [10]. The ascending mental artery can be detected from the extension of the submental artery and when a lingual artery embolism occurs, intraoral necrosis might occur [11]. After Doppler ultrasound detection, perpendicular midline injection is recommended (Fig. 9.7).

Botulinum toxin injection at mentalis muscle can be performed concomitantly (Fig. 9.8).

9.3 Lip Injection

Lip augmentation is a common filler procedure in western countries [12]. Large lips look more attractive in western society. But in Oriental patients, many patients have horizontal long lips, mouth protrusion, and microgenia [13]. So for Oriental patients, the appropriate filler injection needed depends on the harmony of the lips and

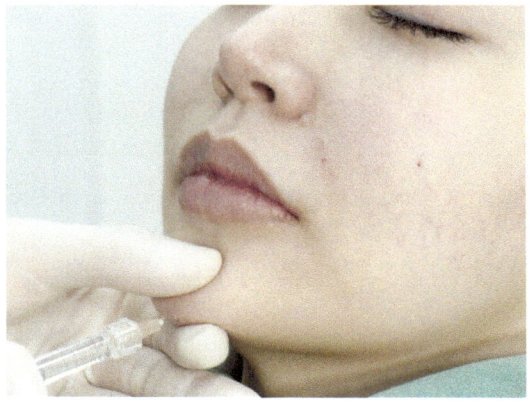

Fig. 9.7 Perpendicular midline injection by needle after detecting submental artery by Doppler ultrasound

face (Fig. 9.9). Appropriate lip augmentation and lip border enhancement can make improvements not only for small lip patients but also for perioral wrinkles from the aging process. The aging process tends to result in loss of lip border and make perioral small wrinkles. Recently, the mouth cor-

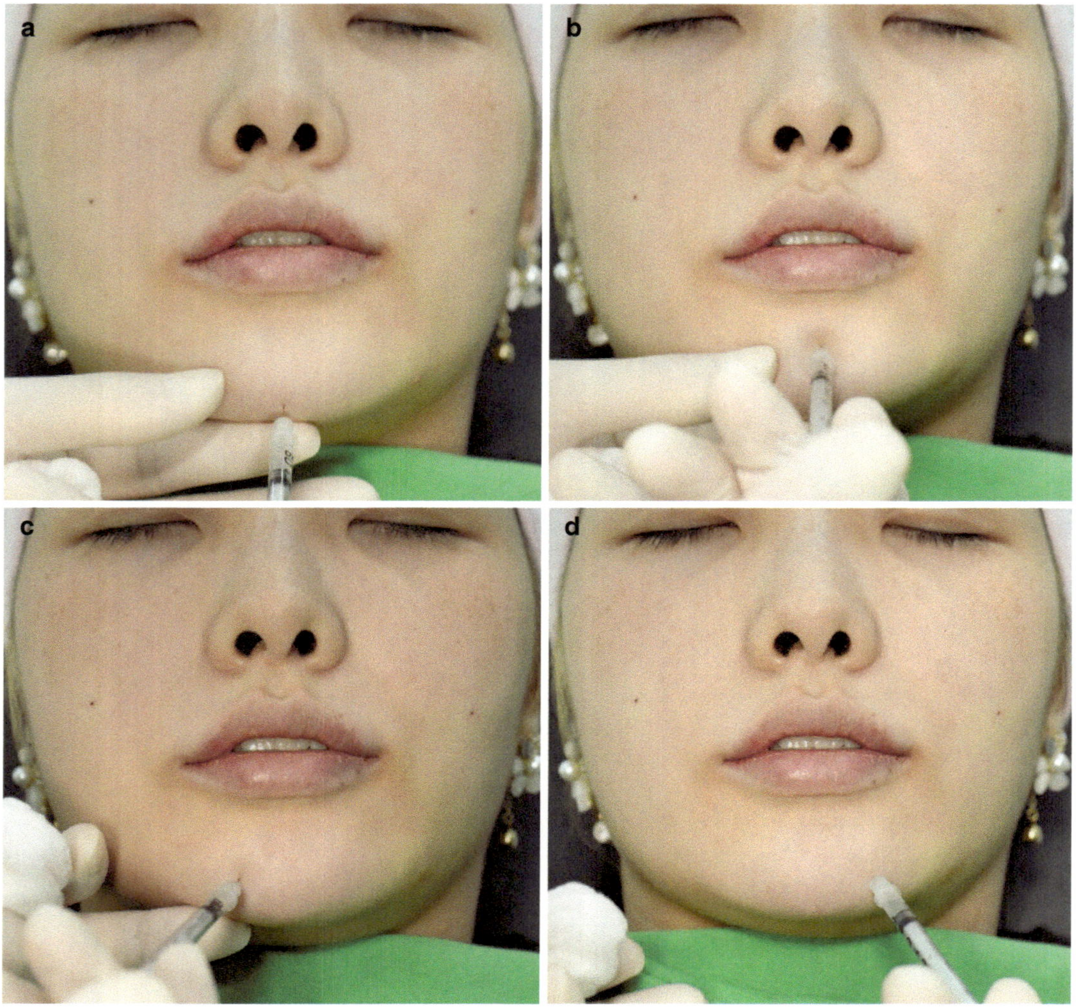

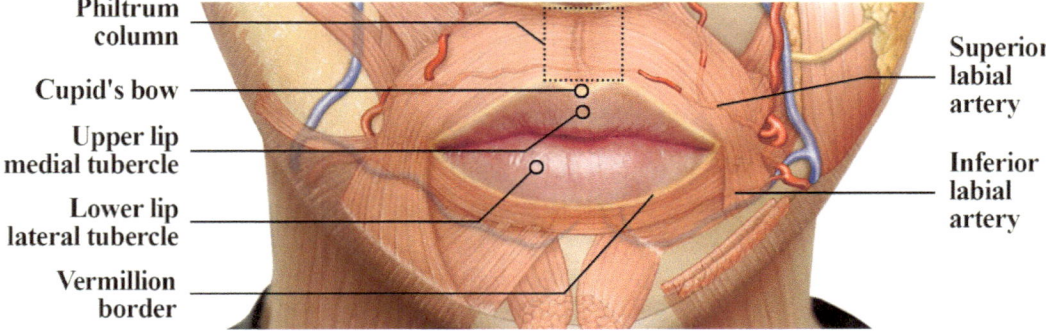

Fig. 9.8 Botulinum toxin injection. (**a**) Lower, (**b**) Upper (deep), (**c**) Right, and (**d**) Left

Philtrum column

Cupid's bow

Upper lip medial tubercle

Lower lip lateral tubercle

Vermillion border

Superior labial artery

Inferior labial artery

Fig. 9.9 Nomenclature of lips

ner lifting process is also commonly performed so a description of border enhancement, augmentation, and mouth corner lifting shall follow in this chapter.

The ideal proportion is 1:1.5. For border enhancement, the patient can lie down but for augmentation, the patient should be in an upright position. Always should consider vascular anatomy (Figs. 9.10 and 9.11).

9.3.1 Anesthesia

Usually performed by topical anesthetic ointment or regional nerve block. A regional nerve block for the upper lip is an infraorbital nerve block (Fig. 9.12) and for the lower lip is the mental nerve block (Fig. 9.13).

9.3.2 Lip Border Enhancement

The vermillion border should be prominent for attractive lips. As the aging process progresses, the lip border becomes more obscure, so border enhancement is needed for young attractive lips.

The injection should be performed from lateral to medial (Fig. 9.14). When injection is vice versa, the filler can ooze to the previous injection point.

9.3.3 Lip Augmentation

Lips, especially the lower lip, are attractive when well padded. Volume augmentation should be

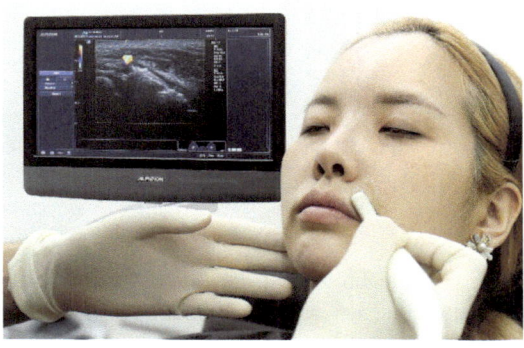

Fig. 9.10 Doppler ultrasound finding of superior labial artery

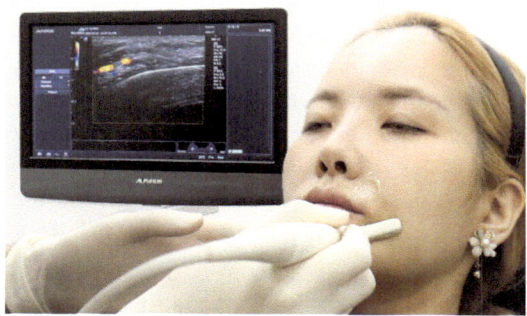

Fig. 9.11 Doppler ultrasound finding of inferior labial artery

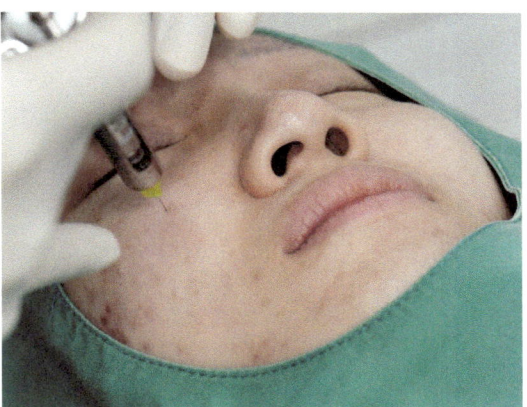

Fig. 9.12 Infraorbital nerve regional block

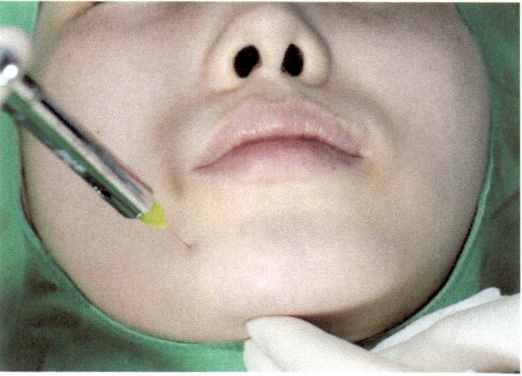

Fig. 9.13 Mental nerve regional block

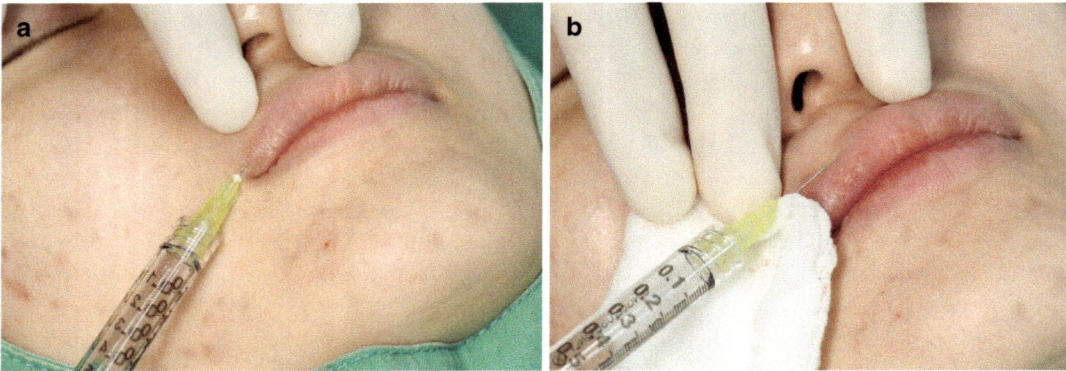

Fig. 9.14 Upper lip border enhancement. (**a**) Starts laterally and (**b**) Moves to medial location

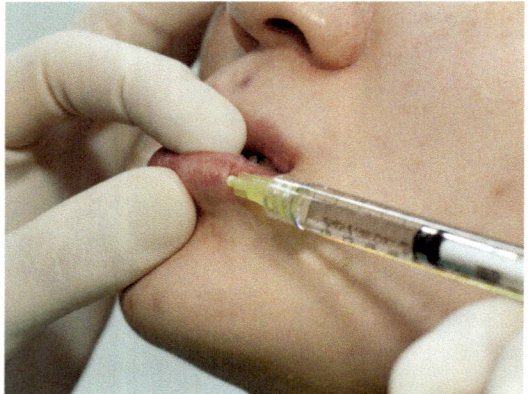

Fig. 9.15 Lower lip augmentation. More volume is needed compare to upper lip

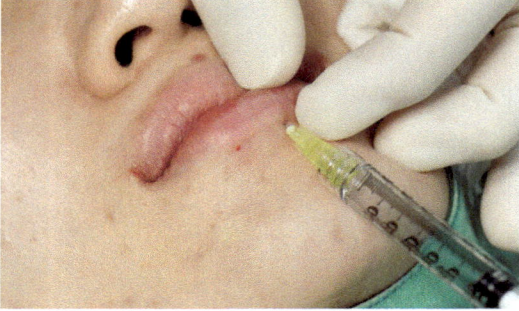

Fig. 9.16 Lower lip lateral tubercle bolus injection

performed for the lower lip (Fig. 9.15). For volume injection, a superficial injection is a better layer than a muscle layer. The superficial labial artery and inferior labial artery run in the mucosal layer so it is relatively safe to inject in the superficial subcutaneous layer.

For lower lip augmentation, a bilateral cherry shape lower tubercle should be considered (Fig. 9.16). Evenly over filling the lip would show sausage lips or duck lips [14]. So a bilateral tubercle enhancement is a useful technique [15]. But since it is a bolus technique, doctors should consider foreign body sensation or granuloma formation.

9.3.4 Mouth Corner Lifting

Recently, many patients desire mouth corner lifting. Mouth corner lifting is a multiple procedure which is to augment the lateral part of the upper lip, support the marionette line and weaken the depressor anguli oris muscle by botulinum toxin [16]. Interestingly, mentalis also affects mouth corner depression so injecting botulinum toxin at the mentalis muscle also should be performed [17].

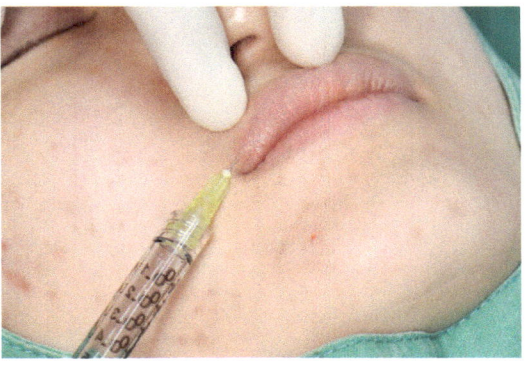

Fig. 9.17 Upper lip lateral side volume augmentation

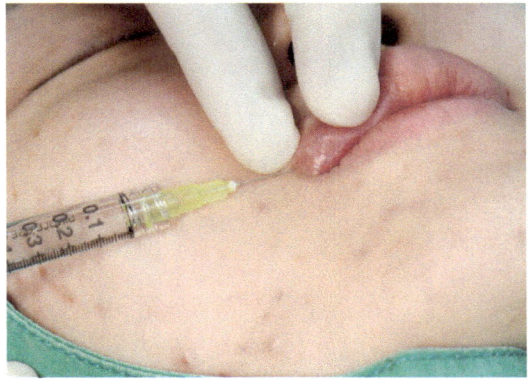

Fig. 9.18 More mucosa should be shown at lateral part of upper lip

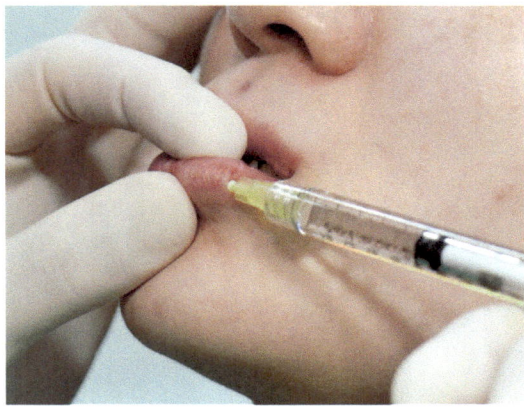

Fig. 9.19 Lower lip volume augmentation

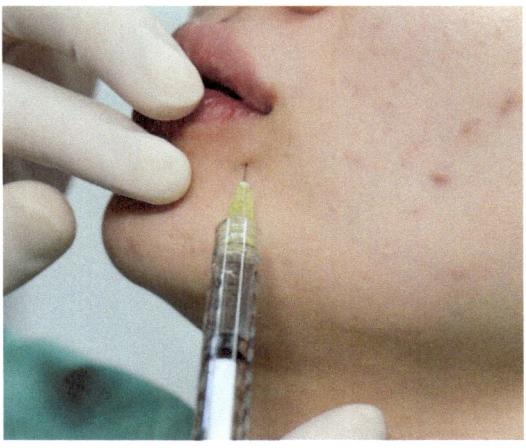

Mouth corner lifting procedure (Figs. 9.17, 9.18, 9.19, 9.20, 9.21, and 9.22).

Fig. 9.20 Upper part of marionette line, 0.1 ~ 0.15 mL of HA filler injected to support mouth corner

9.3.5   Filler Choice

Recently some products named ~ lips have appeared in the market. This means lip augmentation patients are increasing. As I described previously, a lip injection should be performed superficially, and the filler contour and color should be considered. Usually, a low elastic and high cohesive filler is used because lips are a highly movable structure when eating and talking, so a relatively soft filler is used not to feel a foreign body sensation. Lorient No. 2 is used (Table 9.3).

9.3.6   Pre- and Postprocedural Photographs (Figs. 9.23, 9.24, 9.25, and 9.26)

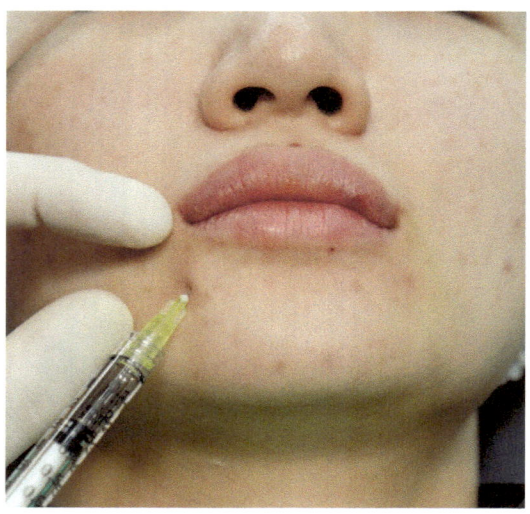

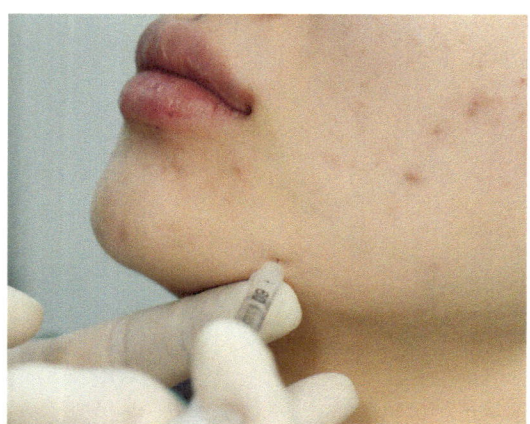

Fig. 9.22 Inject botulinum toxin 4 U ipsilaterally divided into 2 ~ 3 injection sites. Mentalis muscle injection should also be performed (Fig. 9.8)

Fig. 9.21 Inject marionette line with skin stretching for additional mouth corner support

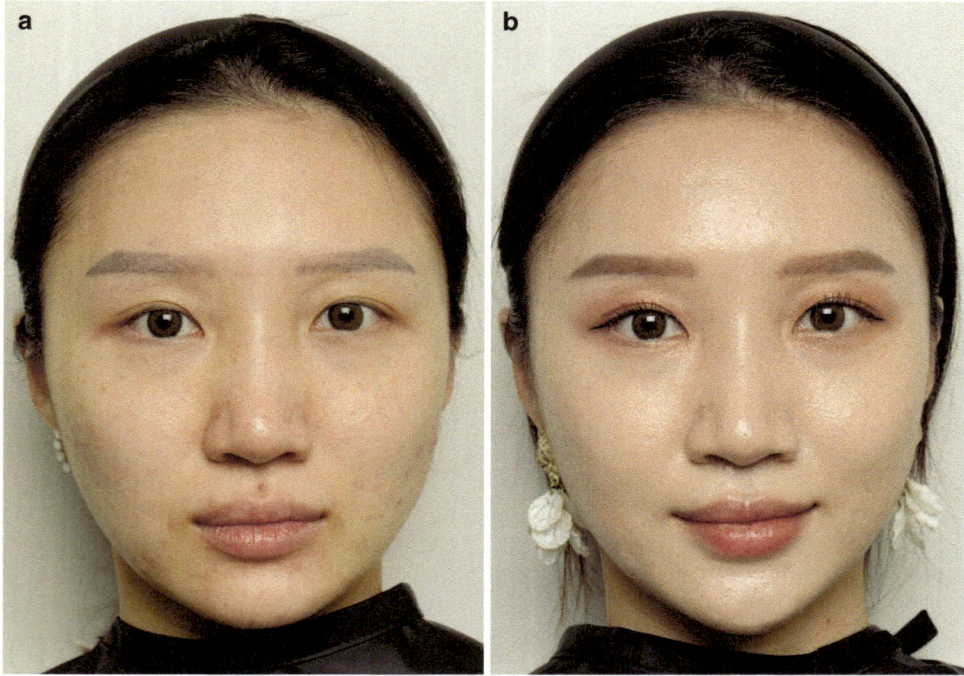

Fig. 9.23 A 29-year-old female patient mouth corner lifting (**a**) preprocedural front view and (**b**) postprocedural 2-week front view. The upper lip left part is depressed so augmentation was also performed

Table 9.3 Rheologic tests for Lorient filler

Product	G′ (Pa)	G″ (Pa)	Complex viscosity (μ)	Tan delta	Cohesiveness (N)
Lorient No. 2	203	41	1,673,007	0.20	0.4401
Lorient No. 4	338	95	2,795,776	0.28	0.4237
Lorient No. 6	413	121	3,423,232	0.29	0.4454

The author uses No. 2 for lips

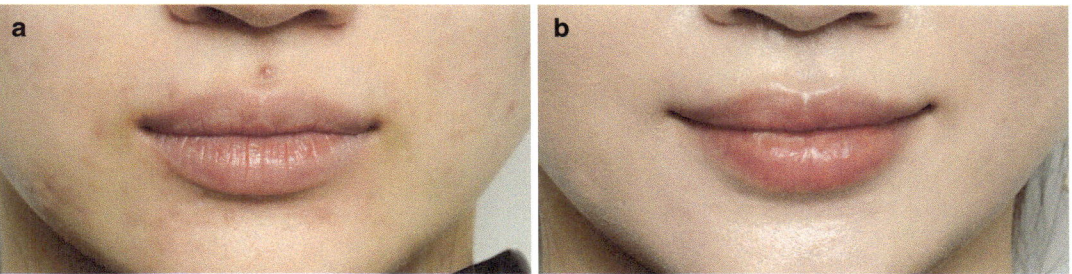

Fig. 9.24 Lips (**a**) pre and (**b**) post close up photograph

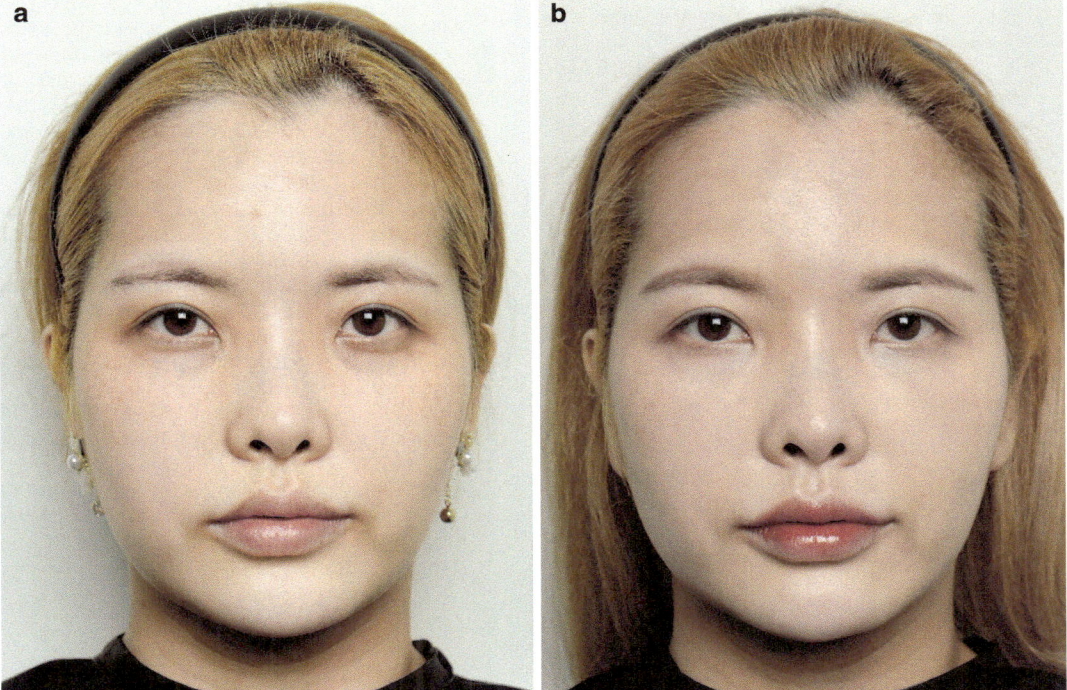

Fig. 9.25 A 29-old-female patient mouth corner lifting (**a**) preprocedural front view and (**b**) postprocedural 2 weeks front view. Tear trough correction was also performed

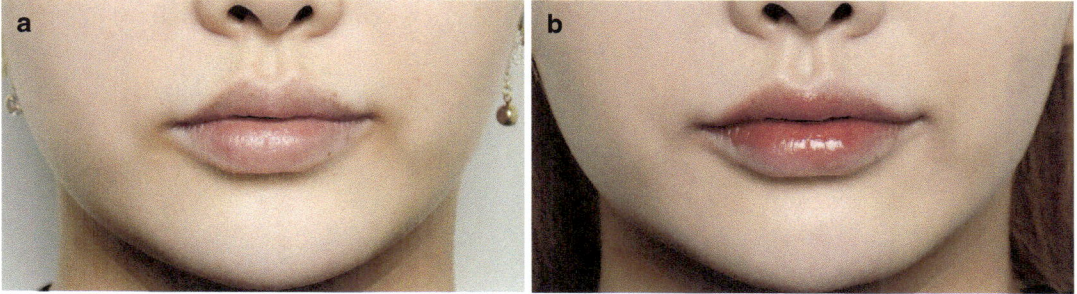

Fig. 9.26 Lips (**a**) pre and (**b**) post close up photograph

References

1. Gierloff M, Stöhring C, Buder T, Wiltfang J. The subcutaneous fat compartments in relation to aesthetically important facial folds and rhytides. J Plast Reconstr Aesthet Surg. 2012 Oct;65(10):1292–7.

2. Braz A, Humphrey S, Weinkle S, Yee GJ, Remington BK, Lorenc ZP, et al. Lower face: clinical anatomy and regional approaches with injectable fillers. Plast Reconstr Surg. 2015;136(5 Suppl):235s–57s.

3. Lee SH, Lee M, Kim HJ. Anatomy-based image processing analysis of the running pattern of the perioral artery for minimally invasive surgery. Br J Oral Maxillofac Surg. 2014 Oct;52(8):688–92.

4. Ricketts RM. Perspectives in the clinical application of cephalometrics. The first fifty years. Angle Orthod. 1981 Apr;51(2):115–50. https://doi.org/10.1043/0003-3219(1981)051<0115:PITCAO>2.0.CO;2.

5. Standring S. Gray's Anatomy. 40th ed. New York: Elsevier/Churchill Livingstone, 2008:484Y488.

6. Hur MS, Kim HJ, Choi BY, Hu KS, Kim HJ, Lee KS. Morphology of the mentalis muscle and its relationship with the orbicularis oris and incisivus labii inferioris muscles. J Craniofac Surg. 2013 Mar;24(2):602–4. https://doi.org/10.1097/SCS.0b013e318267bcc5.

7. Guo X, Zhao J, Song G, Zong X, Zhang D, Lai C, Jin X. Unexpected bone resorption in mentum induced by the soft-tissue filler hyaluronic acid: a preliminary retrospective cohort study of Asian patients. Plast Reconstr Surg. 2020 Aug;146(2):147e–155e. https://doi.org/10.1097/PRS.0000000000006979.

8. Lee W, Yang EJ. Unexpected bone resorption in mentum induced by the soft-tissue filler hyaluronic acid: a preliminary retrospective cohort study of Asian patients. Plast Reconstr Surg. 2021 Jun 1;147(6):1063e–1064e. https://doi.org/10.1097/PRS.0000000000007926.

9. Buckingham ED, Glasgold R, Kontis T, Smith SP Jr, Dolev Y, Fitzgerald R, Lam SM, Williams EF, Pollei TR. Volume rejuvenation of the lower third, perioral, and jawline. Facial Plast Surg. 2015 Feb;31(1):70–9. https://doi.org/10.1055/s-0035-1544945.

10. Wang Q, Zhao Y, Li H, Li P, Wang J. Vascular complications after chin augmentation using hyaluronic acid. Aesthet Plast Surg. 2018 Apr;42(2):553–9. https://doi.org/10.1007/s00266-017-1036-3.

11. Tansatit T, Phumyoo T, Jitaree B, Sawatwong W, Sahraoui YME. Investigation of the presence and variation of the ascending mental artery: conventional dissections and ultrasonographic study. J Cosmet Dermatol. 2019 Dec;18(6):1821–9. https://doi.org/10.1111/jocd.12928.

12. de Maio M, Wu WTL, Goodman GJ, Monheit G, Alliance for the Future of Aesthetics Consensus Committee. Facial assessment and injection guide for botulinum toxin and injectable hyaluronic acid fillers: focus on the lower face. Plast Reconstr Surg. 2017 Sep;140(3):393e–404e. https://doi.org/10.1097/PRS.0000000000003646.

13. Peng JH, Peng HP. Classifications and injection strategy for lip reshaping in Asians. J Cosmet Dermatol. 2020 Oct;19(10):2519–28. https://doi.org/10.1111/jocd.13635.

14. Tonnard PL, Verpaele AM, Bensimon RH. Centrofacial rejuvenation, vol. III. Germany: Thieme. 2008.

15. Sahan A, Funda T. Four-point injection technique for lip augmentation. Acta Dermatovenerol Alp Pannonica Adriat. 2018 Jun;27(2):71–3.

16. Jeong TK. Mouth corner lift with botulinum toxin type a and hyaluronic acid filler. Plast Reconstr Surg. 2020;145(3):538e–41e.

17. Bae GY, Na JI, Park KC, Cho SB. Nonsurgical correction of drooping mouth corners using monophasic hyaluronic acid and incobotulinumtoxinA. J Cosmet Dermatol. 2020;19(2):338–45.